BE HEALTHIER,

Naturally

ROSE TESTA

Printed in the United States of America

ISBN-13: 978-1981146529
ISBN-10: 1981146520

10 9 8 7 6 5 4 3 2

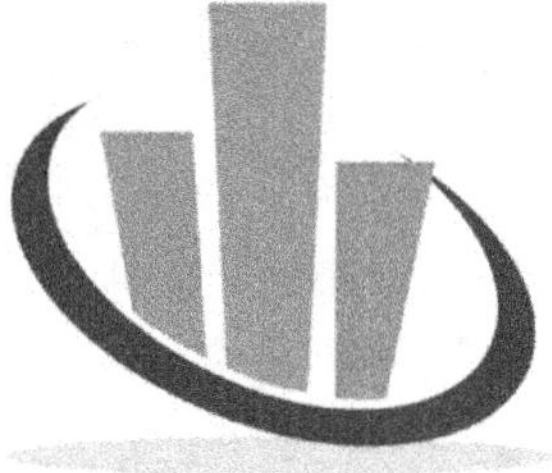

EMPIRE PUBLISHING

www.empirebookpublishing.com

DISCLAIMER

This book is designed to provide helpful information on the subjects discussed. It is not meant to be used to diagnose or treat any medical condition. The reader should consult a physician for diagnosis or treatment of any medical problem. The publisher and author are not responsible for any specific health or allergy issues that may require medical supervision. They are not liable for any damages or negative consequences from any treatment, application or preparation, to any person reading or following the information in this book. References are provided for informational purposes only and do not constitute an endorsement of any websites, products or other sources. Readers should be aware that any websites or products mentioned in this book may change or be discontinued.

DEDICATION

There are many people to thank and for whom I am grateful. The following are among those who generously shared their knowledge and assisted me during my natural education journey. My brother John Howley, Angela Harris and her wonderful family. Becky Boyd, Karen Jackson, Carol Richards, Sari Wilde, RaShelle Roberts and all my amazing Herbie friends along the way. Also, I especially owe a debt of gratitude to my understanding mother and sons, who put up with me and all my experiments!

INTRODUCTION

I'm just a Jersey girl from Atlantic City. Eating pizza, pasta, subs, Italian bread, sugary foods and drinking soda was my basic diet. Healthy eating? What was that?? I never imagined or thought food or what I ate or drank affecting my health.

I was pregnant and had a one year old when my ex left me. I was physically and financially abandoned so I moved to Las Vegas to live with family who had moved there. Having kids made me start thinking about what we eat and maybe eating healthier. I couldn't afford fancy foods or supplements. In fact, my training ground began by trying to provide healthier options via food stamps. During this period, I started learning about the health benefits of garlic, extra virgin olive oil, apple cider vinegar and simply drinking enough water. These changes made me begin to realize that you could really improve your health with a few simple changes. Soon I began learning about whole food blending, bought a Vitamix and began making whole food blender drinks. Guess what happened? Like many people, I progressed and then returned to some bad eating habits again.

After some time, I became a massage therapist and chiropractic assistant and started learning how the body works. Soon after, I added the study of essential oils, stones & crystals, muscle testing, reflexology, ear candling, reiki, how emotions affect our health and a little bit of knowledge about herbs. I started using what I learned on my family, friends, clients and me. I was taking synthetic vitamins and thought I would see a huge improvement, but I was disappointed to see I didn't get the results I wanted.

I had a skin cancer scare which made me think about investigating more deeply into the healing properties of herbs. I began taking classes at a newly opened local herbal health food store, Herbally Grounded, and I began researching once again. I also began experiencing menopause symptoms and decided to try herbs to balance my hormones. I had no idea my hormones were out of balance until I found myself thinking clearer, having more patience, feeling calmer and sleeping better without having to use the standard treatment of drugs, artificial hormones or bioidenticals impressed me. I also started taking powdered greens to replace the synthetic vitamins. I started thinking that everyone needs to know about this approach to health! I thought combining more herbal knowledge with my practice of massage therapy would be an excellent way to help other people. I began an herbal apprenticeship that started at Herbally Grounded. I worked part-time at the store and was able to research and absorb an enormous variety of information; I was particularly intrigued to learn how our face and body show us symptoms of health problems. During all this process, I slowly continued to make more natural changes in my life. I began making my own herbal remedies followed by making personal care, bath and cleaning products and I continue to experiment and learn and try all kinds of new ideas and approaches.

Because of these experiences in my life, I find the natural approach to healthier living the best way to face ailments and physical limitations in life. I believe modern medicine has a wonderful place in our society to help with emergencies, broken bones, testing and so forth. However, I think that we are all aware that medications can present problems such as side effects that cause other health issues and each person differs; some may not do well on a medication that many others tolerate well. Many articles point out that we are living longer today than previously in history. We certainly have better sanitation knowledge, refrigeration, and indoor plumbing & sewer systems. We also have better methods of transportation to offer access to a wide availability of healthier food options.

I also have benefited from having my blood tested to determine what issues I might need to address. I found that my blood sugar and cholesterol levels were high. Of course, medication was recommended. I preferred my own approach because I knew that I could most directly evaluate the effects on my body. I decided to make a number of lifestyle changes such as eating more vegetables and fruits while avoiding sugars and carbs and taking specific herbs known to help maintain healthier blood sugar levels. I also drank whole food blender drinks, bentonite clay water, lemon water and herbal teas. Additionally, I looked at the physical and etheric body health by adding light physical activities, meditation and massages. I mention all these aspects of my treatment because, as you see, natural approaches allow you to experiment and adapt an integral approach to health: mind, body and spirit. Prescription drugs can certainly be chosen, but I felt, particularly after this experience, that if an individual did not change the habits and lifestyle which caused the problem, medications might just mask the symptoms.

Start simple by eating a little healthier and drinking enough water. As you read on, you don't have to try everything listed. Try suggestions that you already have on hand or a few that draw your attention and which feel good to you. I think you should take for at least a week to a month to evaluate your progress and the effects of your changes. Then try something else. Please remember that I give some of my favorite ideas and examples of products as suggestions. You should keep your mind open because you may encounter another idea or product to solve a problem. When using any product, please use them as directed on the label or I might mention other suggestions. I also want you to remember another equally important fact; something that works for you, may not work for others; everyone's body is different. You may not receive an intended effect from an herbal concoction or supplement. That's ok. Try something else. You may discover later, after changing something subtle in your body, that the herb or supplement which didn't work for you on one occasion will work for you on another.

This book is about the things I've learned from my studies, classes, seminars, online research, experiments, personal experiences, along with shared information from all my great herbie friends and natural healer acquaintances. I provided short basic descriptions or explanations for some of the information provided. If something interests you or you need more information, please do some more research on your own. I'm sharing this information with you so you can become aware of some symptoms and causes of health issues before they become severe. I'm hoping this information will encourage you to re-evaluate your lifestyle and begin some changes if you need to do so. So many issues can be reversed. Pay attention to what your body tells you! Take control of your health, and if you have a health issue, don't panic. Most of the symptoms listed are warning signs, and the body is infinitely adaptable. You're not expected to change overnight, simply do the best you can. You may feel like changing a health habit is too much work, or you may get off track sometimes, but guess what? You're human. The important idea to keep in mind is that you will simply try again, or try something different on your journey to getting healthier.

Here's to your good health!!

TABLE OF CONTENTS

BE HEALTHIER,

Naturally

HERBS

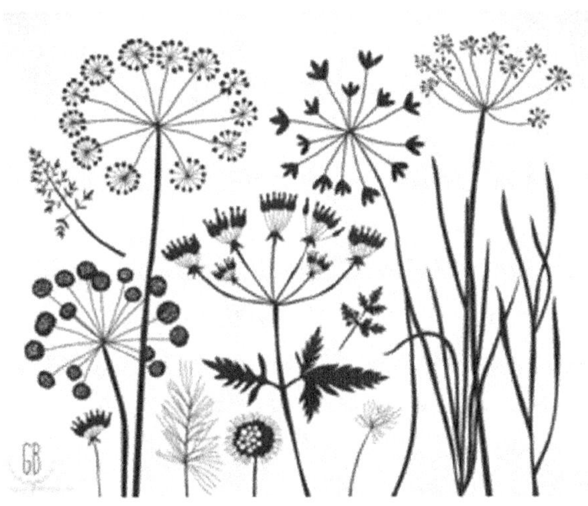

BASIS OF HEALTH

HOW TO MAKE & USE HERBAL REMEDIES

Herbs are grasses, weeds, spices, leaves, seeds, berries, flowers or any other plant materials, which are mostly used for their medicinal properties, cooking or aromatherapy. Herbs should be stored in airtight containers away from sunlight and extreme heat. They are a natural way to get nutrition and to cleanse and rebuild our bodies. Herbs are food, so our body will recognize and absorb the nutrition from them more efficiently as opposed to taking synthetic products.

Herbs have been safely used medicinally in all cultures throughout history. Herbal remedies have proven to be very effective and remain so. Unfortunately, somewhere around the 1920's, the pharmaceutical industry started taking over, and a new mindset kicked in. I'm grateful people are becoming more aware again, of the benefits of natural healing, instead of using pharmaceuticals. Hippocrates is known as the "Father of Medicine." He did not use penicillin or insulin but used herbal remedies as medicine.

You can grow your own herbs. I'm not much of a gardener so I like to buy my herbs, dried or powdered, by the ounce from health food stores, online herbal suppliers and you can also buy herbs at many grocery stores.

Before you start any DIY recipe; you should clean and sanitize preparation tools. Sanitizing helps prevent contamination and allows the DIY product to last longer. Soak all preparation tools such as empty bottles, jars, bowls, droppers, funnels and utensils in a bowl with hydrogen peroxide or rubbing alcohol for a few minutes and let them dry completely. You can also put hydrogen peroxide or rubbing alcohol in a spray bottle and spray preparation tools, jars and containers and let them dry completely before using. Remember to label all containers with product name, and maybe the date made and list of ingredients.

Determining Your Herbal Combination or Formula - you can take an individual herb by itself or choose herbs that work together in addressing your health issue. Let's use someone wanting to improve their liver function. They could use a combination of like herbs that are known to strengthen your liver (e.g., barberry, dandelion and olive leaf). Equal parts can be used, or if you feel you need more of one or another after reading and research, simply use higher amounts.

Here are herbal combination examples:
- **Good Mood Combination** - 2 parts borage, 3 parts rhodiola rosea and 5 parts St. John's Wort.
- **Vitamin C Combination** - equal parts of each: acerola, amla berry, camu camu and rosehips.

Encapsulation (make your own herbal pill supplements) - encapsulate your own single powdered herb or powdered herbal combination. Buy your own encapsulating machine like *The Capsule Machine* and empty capsules to fill and make your own pills. Instructions come with the machine and are very easy. Empty capsules come in gelatin or vegetarian form and in different size lots: O, OO and OOO. Be sure to get the same size capsules to go with encapsulating machine. Average adult dose is usually 1 to 4 capsules, depending on size of the capsules or adult and take pills with a full glass of water.

When buying pill supplements look for products that don't contain a lot of unnatural fillers or "other ingredients". Don't be afraid to take different herbs or combinations at the same time. Herbs are just dried ground up food. Since herbs are not a drug, it's not much different than eating an apple and a banana at the same time.

HERBAL BLEND OR SINGLE HERB TEA/INFUSION

Herbal teas are hot beverages made using a single herb or making an herbal combination tea. They are mostly consumed for their medicinal effects. You can buy herbal tea combinations at most grocery stores or make your own herbal combination.

My Favorite Dried Nutritious Herbal Tea Combination
- Alfalfa Leaf
- Chamomile Flower
- Green Stevia Leaf
- Hawthorn Leaf
- Hibiscus Flower
- Moringa Leaf
- Mullein Leaf
- Nettle Leaf
- Peppermint Leaf
- Red Raspberry Leaf

Use all above ingredients or any above dried herbal combination. Mix ingredients together and store in closed container.

How to Make Hot Herbal Tea
- Put about 1 teaspoon to 1 tablespoon of herbal tea combination into a cup, a small tea ball, mesh tea strainer, canning jar infuser or make tea bags with small press n' brew empty tea bags.
- Place herbs into cup or mug; fill cup with boiling water and steep for about 10 to 20 minutes. If using roots, stems or seeds, steep a bit longer.
- Optional to add some fresh lemon juice, lemon slices, lemon zest, orange zest, cinnamon, raw honey, agave, flavored stevia extract, green stevia or peppermint leaves.

Decoction - a strong herbal tea. By using heat, this is a good way to extract nutrition from roots, seeds and stems.

Example - **Yellow Dock Root Decoction Recipe**
- Put 2 ounces of cut dried yellow dock root into a quart glass jar with a lid.
- Fill with boiling filtered or distilled water.
- Cover and let steep for 8 hours or overnight.
- Empty into a glass, enamel or stainless steel pan (not aluminum) and heat on low temperature for 20 to 30 minutes.

- Let cool and strain decoction through muslin cloth, muslin bag, cheesecloth or coffee filter, and squeeze out as much liquid as possible from roots.
- Optional to add ¼ cup blackstrap molasses or brandy to sweeten the liquid if desired.
- Store in refrigerator; take 1 to 3 tablespoons daily. Consume until gone and should be enough for about 2 weeks.
- Rebuilds iron levels and blood purifier.
- Acts as a laxative and aids digestion.

HERBAL TINCTURE/EXTRACT

A tincture/extract is a liquid herbal remedy made with glycerin & distilled water, apple cider vinegar or alcohol as a base ingredient.

How to Make Glycerin & Distilled Water Tincture - food grade vegetable glycerin is a thick liquid that is colorless and sweet tasting. It metabolizes more slowly in the body, so it's not known to have a dramatic effect on blood sugar levels. Good to look for kosher certified USP grade and non-GMO.

Ingredients:
- 2 parts food grade vegetable glycerin
- 2 parts distilled water
- 1 part powdered herb(s) or 2 part cut dried herb(s)

How to Make
- Put all ingredients in canning jar or glass jar with a lid, shake or stir to mix.
- Cover, label and date. Keep jar on counter or in cabinet; let steep for about 2 weeks, shake or stir 1 to 2 times a day.
- When tincture is ready, strain liquid through muslin cloth, muslin bag, cheesecloth or coffee filter by hand into bowl, or use a tincture press.
- Pour extracted liquid preferably into a dark glass dropper bottles.
- Store the remaining liquid in a glass jar in the refrigerator.

Example - **Red Raspberry Glycerin Tincture**
- 1 cup food grade vegetable glycerin
- 1 cup distilled water
- 1 cup cut dried red raspberry leaf or ½ cup red raspberry powder

How to Make Apple Cider Vinegar or Alcohol Tincture - use raw unfiltered apple cider vinegar or alcohol (e.g., vodka, rum or brandy)

Ingredients:
- 4 parts apple cider vinegar or alcohol
- 1 part powdered herb(s) or 2 parts cut dried herb(s)

How to Make
- Put all ingredients in canning jar or glass jar with a lid, shake or stir to mix.
- Cover, label and date. Keep jar on counter or in cabinet; let steep for about 2 weeks; shake or stir 1 to 2 times a day.
- When tincture is ready, strain liquid through muslin cloth, muslin bag, cheesecloth or coffee filter by hand into bowl, or use a tincture press.
- Pour extracted liquid preferably into a dark glass dropper bottles.
- Store the remaining liquid in a glass jar in the refrigerator.

Example - **Milk Thistle Seed Apple Cider Vinegar Tincture**
- 1 cup apple cider vinegar
- ¼ cup milk thistle seed powder

How to take tinctures - average adult dose is 3 squirts which equals about 1 teaspoon & take 1 to 3 times a day:
- By mouth or under the tongue.
- In water, juice, coconut water or warm herbal tea.
- Foods like applesauce, yogurt, pudding and oatmeal.

Children take lesser amounts of herbs:
- Up to 1 year - ⅙ of adult dosage
- Years 1 to 6 - ⅓ of adult dosage
- 6 to 12 - ½ of adult dosage

HERBAL OIL & SALVE, OINTMENT

Herbal oil is a carrier oil infused with an herb's essence, and a salve/ointment is herbal oil thickened by adding wax. Some uses for herbal oils and salves include moisturizing skin and treating any number of conditions including cuts, burns, scrapes, insect bites, chapped lips, sunburn, rashes, scars, itching, stretch marks and much more.

Carrier Oils - are known as base oils, usually derived from vegetable fats, nuts or seeds. You should buy oils that are 100% oil with no fragrances or preservatives (simply cold pressed oil). Carrier oils are used to make DIY recipes including herbal oils, herbal salves, body oils, facial oils, creams and lotions. They are also used to dilute essential oils before they are applied to skin.

Some Good Carrier Oil Choices

- Almond Oil
- Apricot Kernel Oil
- Argan Oil
- Avocado Oil
- Baobab Oil
- Calendula Oil
- Coconut Oil
- Emu Oil
- Evening Primrose Oil
- Extra Virgin Olive Oil
- Grapeseed Oil
- Hazelnut Oil
- Hemp Oil
- Jojoba Oil
- Macadamia Oil
- Moringa Oil
- Mustard Seed Oil
- Pumpkin Seed Oil
- Red Raspberry Seed Oil
- Rosehip Oil
- Safflower Oil
- Sesame Seed Oil
- Sunflower Oil
- Walnut Oil

HERBAL OIL

Ingredients:
- 3 to 4 parts carrier oil(s)
- 1 part herb(s) - dried or powdered

How to Make Basic Herbal Oil in Canning Jar
- Fill canning jar or glass jar with a lid about ⅓ full with dried herb(s) or ¼ full with powdered herb(s).

- Fill up jar with carrier oil(s) of your choice, shake or stir to mix together.
- Cover, label and date.
- Keep jar on counter or in cabinet.
- Let steep for about 2 weeks; shake or stir 1 to 2 times a day; the longer you steep, the stronger the oil.
- When oil is ready, strain oil through muslin cloth, muslin bag, cheesecloth or coffee filter by hand into a bowl, or use a tincture press.
- Pour extracted oil into bottles.
- Optional - after straining, you can stir in essential oils before putting into bottles.

Herbal Oil in Canning Jar

Example - **Chaparral Oil**

- Fill jar ⅓ full with dried chaparral leaves or ¼ full with chaparral powder.
- Then, fill up of jar with ½ extra virgin olive oil & grapeseed oil.
- Cover, label and date; after 2 weeks of shaking daily, strain oil.
- Add 5 drops each of clove, oregano & tea tree essential oils to strained oil.
- Some uses include athlete's foot, bites, burns, cold sores, dandruff, eczema, fungus, lice, psoriasis, rashes, wounds, toenail or any fungal skin infection.

Herbal Oil in Crock-pot

Example - **Lavender Oil**

- In small crock-pot on warm or low setting.
- ⅓ cup dried flowers or ¼ cup powdered with 1 cup any carrier oil.
- Stir, cover and steep for 1 to 7 days; stir a few times a day; the longer you steep, the stronger the oil.
- The heat from crock-pot will extract essence from herbs faster than the above jar recipe.
- When oil is ready, strain oil through muslin cloth, muslin bag, cheesecloth or coffee filter by hand into bowl, or use a tincture press.
- Pour extracted oil into bottles.
- Optional - after straining, you can add essential oils before putting into bottles.
- Some uses include skin moisturizer, wrinkles, bites, burns, sunburns, rashes and wounds.

HERBAL SALVE

Ingredients:
- 3 parts herbal oil of choice
- 1 part beeswax (vegan alternative is carnauba wax)

How to Make Herbal Salve in Crock-pot
- Heat herbal oil & melt beeswax in small crock-pot.
- Once melted & blended, turn crock-pot off to cool some.
- Pour warm liquid salve into jars to harden. If using plastic containers, be careful oil is not too hot or your containers could melt.
- Start by filling only one jar to harden to test the consistency of salve. If too hard, put back into crock-pot and add some herbal oil; if it is too loose, add some more wax.

ESSENTIAL OILS

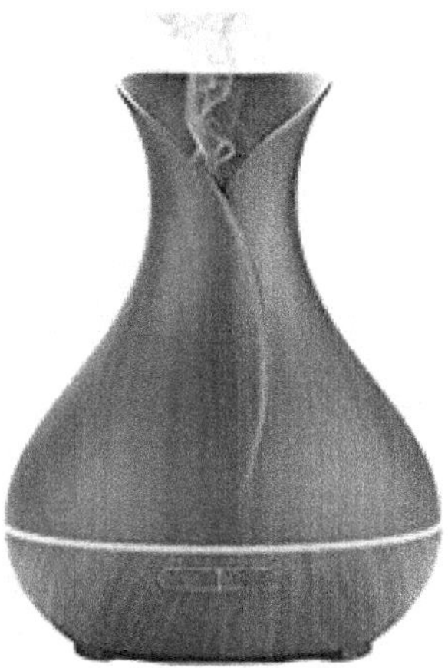

Essential oils have been used for thousands of years. The Greeks, Romans, Native Indians and ancient Egyptians all used essential oils in their spiritual practices, healing rituals, perfumes, baths and massages. In 1910, French chemist Rene-Maurice Gattefosse first discovered the benefits of lavender essential oil when he had a laboratory accident and set his arm on fire. He put his arm into the nearest liquid, which happened to be a vat of lavender essential oil. Almost immediately, he noticed some pain relief and his wound healed quickly without infection or scarring. He experimented during the First World War with clove, lavender, lemon and thyme essential oils for their antiseptic properties and saw wounds heal faster.

When essential oils are inhaled, the smell travels across the olfactory nerves, into the brain which controls our moods, fears, memories and ability to learn. This is our limbic system and when stimulated, our body will release endorphins and other "feel good" chemicals. Smells have a subtle way of affecting your mind and emotions. We all have times when we smell something which triggers a childhood memory or maybe the smell of a friend's house.

Some of the Various Benefits Associated With the Following Essential Oils

- **Basil** - respiratory issues, calming, nausea, motion sickness and digestion.
- **Bergamot** - antidepressant, uplifts spirits, feel calmer, brings hope, attracts money and success.

- **Birch** - antibacterial, anti-inflammatory, decongestant, respiratory issues, digestion, sore muscles and joints and helps balance mood swings.
- **Black Pepper** - digestion, sore muscles and joints, stress, promotes courage and emotional strength and clears negative energy.
- **Carrot Seed** - sunscreen protection, dry skin, lines, wrinkles, eczema, psoriasis, liver spots and helps let go of past mistakes.
- **Cedarwood** - anti-inflammatory, expectorant, insect repellant, wounds, acne, sore muscles and joints.
- **Chamomile** - anti-inflammatory, antidepressant, nerve sedative, calming, relaxing, headaches, motion sickness, attracts good luck and money.
- **Cinnamon** - antibacterial, antiparasitic, benefits hormones, acne, digestion, oral health, attracts money, love and success.
- **Citronella** - anti-fungal, anti-inflammatory, antidepressant, insect repellent, uplifts spirits, anxiety and promotes hope.
- **Clary Sage** - antidepressant, uplifts spirits, stress, benefits adrenals and hormones, menopause, grounding and helps clear negative energy.
- **Clove** - antibacterial, antifungal, antiviral, oral health, athlete's foot, heavy metals, promotes healing, attracts money and drives away harmful forces.
- **Cypress** - wound healer, respiratory issues, anxiety, go with the flow, grounding and helps let go of past mistakes.
- **Davana** - antiviral, wound healer, relaxing, benefits hormones, uplifts spirits, stress and anxiety.
- **Eucalyptus** - anti-inflammatory, decongestant, respiratory issues, coughs, sore muscles and joints, staph infection, shingles, insect repellant, purifies and clears room of negative conflict.
- **Frankincense** - anti-inflammatory, respiratory issues, enhance meditations, stimulates brain function, improves memory, soothing effect on mind and enhances intuition.
- **Geranium** - wound healer, benefits adrenals and hormones, menopause, uplifts spirits, insect repellent, breaks hexes and blessing the new.
- **Ginger** - anti-inflammatory, expectorant, analgesic, motion sickness, nausea, digestion, sore muscles and joints and attracts money.
- **Grapefruit** - antidepressant, antibacterial, suppresses appetite, uplifts spirits, benefits hormones, clears negative energy, releases blame, anger and self-criticism.
- **Helichrysum** - anti-inflammatory, expectorant, analgesic, sore muscles and joints, nerve sedative, wound healer, burns, sunscreen protection, enhances creativity, intuition and opens up the heart.

- **Jasmine** - antidepressant, benefits hormones, increases libido, calming, relaxing, anxiety, uplifts spirits, attracts love and strengthens imagination.
- **Juniper Berry** - anti-inflammatory, wound healer, digestion, helps release fears, insecurities and anger.
- **Lavender** - antifungal, anti-inflammatory, calming, relaxing, stimulates brain function, benefits hormone, acne, stress, sunscreen protection, burns, sunburn, insect repellent, uplifts spirits, enhance meditations, attracts love, promotes peace at home and lightens energy when we are agitated or over excited.
- **Lemon** - antiviral, disinfectant, antibacterial, stimulates lymphatic drainage, wrinkles, shingles, oral health, digestion, nausea, uplifts spirits, and can get rid of sticky goo residue.
- **Lemon Balm** - wound healer, digestion, benefits thyroid, headaches, anxiety, calming, relaxing and cold sores.
- **Lemongrass** - antidepressant, uplifts spirits, insect repellent and stimulates psychic awareness.
- **Marjoram** - antibacterial, antiviral, expectorant, wound healer, sore muscles and joints, digestion, benefits hormones, helps to accept and love ourselves.
- **Myrrh** - antifungal, anti-inflammatory, expectorant, wound healer, cold sores, shingles, oral health, expands awareness, calms fears about the future and stimulates psychic awareness.
- **Neem** - antibacterial, wound healer, dry itchy skin, acne, wrinkles, insect repellant, helps with skin pigmentation, vitiligo and liver spots.
- **Neroli** - antidepressant, uplifts spirits, grief, calming, relaxing, attracts money and success.
- **Nutmeg** - analgesic, antibacterial, diarrhea, digestion, attracts money, good luck and breaks evil hexes.
- **Orange** - antidepressant, anti-inflammatory, calming, appetite suppressant, uplifts spirits, benefits hormones, gets rid of sticky goo residue and attracts love and money.
- **Oregano** - antifungal, antibacterial, antiviral, anti-inflammatory, candida, cold sores, oral health and helps to accomplish goals.
- **Patchouli** - antidepressant, nausea, digestion, stress, relaxes the mind and promotes clarity.
- **Peppermint** - decongestant, analgesic, respiratory issues, stimulates brain function, digestion, nausea, motion sickness, sore muscles and joints, halt negative thoughts and brings positive movement in your life.
- **Pine** - antibacterial, respiratory issues, sore muscles and joints, attracts money, grounding, helps to let go and not obsess over past mistakes.

- **Ravensara** - antibacterial, antiviral, antifungal, antidepressant, respiratory issues, shingles, sore muscles and joints, headaches and uplifts spirits.
- **Rose** - antidepressant, grief, calming, benefits hormones, unconditional love, harmony, and attracts love.
- **Rosemary** - anti-inflammatory, antibacterial, analgesic, sore muscles and joints, stimulates brain function, improves memory, hair and scalp, insect repellant and used to enhance intuition.
- **Sage** - antifungal, antibacterial, benefits hormones, menopause, hair and scalp, uplifts spirits, calming and clears negative energy.
- **Sandalwood** - antibacterial, antiviral, anti-inflammatory, stimulates brain function, benefits hormones, attracts love, very calming and relaxing.
- **Spruce** - antifungal, expectorant, respiratory issues, sore muscles and joints, anxiety, benefits hormones and thyroid, attracts money and grounding.
- **Tea Tree or Melaleuca** - antibacterial, antiviral, expectorant, acne, wounds, chickenpox, staph infection, cold sores, foot fungus, strep, insect repellant, eliminates confusion and helps face situations head on.
- **Thula** - expectorant, skin tags, warts, mole and insect repellant.
- **Thyme** - antibacterial, antifungal, expectorant, athlete's foot, respiratory issues, insect repellant, acne, oral health and benefits hormones.
- **Wintergreen** - anti-inflammatory, analgesic, respiratory issues, sore muscles and joints, develops trust, release old beliefs and habits.
- **Ylang Ylang** - antidepressant, lifts spirits, benefits hormones, increases libido, stimulates the senses, attracts love, self-forgiveness, promotes positive emotions and self-confidence.

Some of My Favorite Uses of Essential Oils

- **Aromatherapy Bath Salts** - mix 2 cups of any sea salt with 10 to 15 drops of essential oils of your choice. Keep in closed container; add ½ cup to 1 cup to bath water or 2 to 5 tablespoons to foot bath for about 15 to 45 minutes. As an example, using lavender bath salts can be very relaxing and helps with jetlag when you get to destination.
- **Aromatherapy Oil** - mix together 1 ounce any carrier oil with 5 to 8 drops of essential oils of your choice. Some uses include massage oil, body oil or bath oil.
- **Carpet Aromatherapy** - mix together 1 cup of baking soda or bentonite clay with 15 to 30 drops of essential oils like lemon, lime, orange,

peppermint or lavender. Sprinkle on your rugs, leave on for about 30 minutes and vacuum.

- **Flea Collar** - mix together ½ cup of fresh rosemary tea with 20 to 30 drops of essential oils like cedarwood, geranium, lavender, lemongrass, neem, peppermint, rosemary or tea tree. Cut a piece of string or rope to fit pet's neck and moisten in the tea & essential oils. Roll the rope up in a bandana or handkerchief. Then, tie it around the neck of your pet. Will need to be done at least weekly. Massage the rest of the tea onto your pet's body.
- **Insect Repellant Spray** (2 to 4 ounce spray bottle) - put 1 to 3 tablespoons apple cider vinegar into bottle and fill with half witch hazel & lavender tea. Add 10 to 20 drops of essential oils like citronella, eucalyptus, garlic, lemongrass, lavender, neem, rosemary or tea tree. Spray on clothes, skin and hair.
- **Roll-on** (1 ounce bottle or smaller) - put 5 to 15 drops of essential oils of your choice into bottle and fill with carrier oil with not much of a scent such as safflower, sunflower, grapeseed or jojoba oil. As an example - use a 0.33 ounce roll-on bottle filled with 10 drops of jasmine essential oil & fill with sunflower oil. Some uses include perfume, lip oil or cuticle oil.
- **Sanitizing Air Freshener Spray** (4 ounce spray bottle) - put 5 to 10 drops each of clove, lemon, tea tree and thyme essential oils into spray bottle and fill with distilled water. Some uses include freshening the air or sanitizing your hands and objects such as doorknobs, mattresses and furniture. Also use on wounds, rashes and skin infections.

Aromatherapy Uses of Essential Oils

Essential oils can freshen and cleanse the air where you live, work and drive.

Try adding a few drops to:

- Atomizer Diffuser
- Car Diffuser
- Computer USB Diffuser
- Light Bulb Ring
- Nebulizer Diffuser
- Potpourri
- Ultrasonic Diffuser
- Wall Plug In Diffuser

Crock-pot aromatherapy can infuse a home or work place. Put crock-pot on low or warm setting and fill halfway with water. Add 5 to 15 drops of essential oils such as clove, cinnamon, mints or citrus essential oils. You can also add a few whole cloves, cinnamon sticks, fresh or dried cranberries, peppermint leaves, rosemary leaves, sage leaves, allspice, mulling spices, drops of vanilla and slices or rinds of apples, lemons, limes or oranges. Create your own blend.

Consider the Following When Using Essential Oils
- Look for 100% essential oils.
- For optimal shelf life, keep your essential oils in airtight dark glass bottles. Glass bottles are better since plastic bottles can deteriorate damaging the quality of essential oils.
- Keep oils away from direct sunlight, extreme heat, eye area, and don't put directly into ears.
- Store in a safe place out of reach of children and pets.
- Use sparingly since essential oils are highly concentrated. If left open, oils could dissipate.
- Do not put undiluted essential oils directly into bath water since they will float on top of the water, which might cause discomfort or burning to skin. The best approach would be mixing the essential oil with a carrier oil, sea salt, honey or milk before adding to bath water.
- Look for a high quality therapeutic grade if you plan on taking the essential oil internally and do so with caution.

SOME HEALTHIER CHOICES, IDEAS & SUGGESTIONS

The following is an introduction to some of my favorite products, foods & natural healing information I have learned on my journey to getting healthier.

APPLE CIDER VINEGAR

Apple cider vinegar is fermented juice from crushed apples. Best to get raw, unfiltered, organic, cold pressed apple cider vinegar with the mother (the cloudy formation that settles at the bottom), which contains raw enzymes and gut friendly bacteria. There are suggestions for internal & external uses throughout book.

Contains
Vitamins B6,C and biotin, calcium, folate, hydrochloric acid, iron, magnesium, malic acid, niacin, pantothenic acid, pectin, phosphorus, potassium and sodium.

Internal Benefits
- Has antiviral, antifungal, antibacterial, antibiotic, anti-inflammatory and antiseptic properties.
- Is known to curb appetite and boost energy.
- Reduces inflammation, pain and leg cramps to help against arthritis, bursitis and joint pain.
- Breaks down fat and blocks fat formation.
- Helps strengthen immune system and cleanses lymph nodes.
- Gently removes toxins and calcium deposits from the muscles and cells of the body to help strengthen muscles.
- Aids in maintaining healthier blood sugar, blood pressure and cholesterol levels.
- Helps harmonize the pH alkaline balance.

How to Take Apple Cider Vinegar Internally
- Apple cider vinegar drink - 1 tablespoon each of apple cider vinegar and raw honey in glass of warm water; stir and drink 1 to 3 times a day.
- Mix 1 tablespoon vinegar in glass of water or juice and drink 1 to 3 times a day.

- Burns fat naturally - add 1 tablespoon to 4 ounces of water and drink before each meal.
- Don't forget your pets - add 1 to 2 teaspoons to pet's water for nutrition and controlling fleas.

Some External Uses
- Antiseptic spray - put 1 part apple cider vinegar and 3 parts water in a spray bottle to use on wounds, cutting boards, kitchen surfaces, bathroom surfaces and clean produce.
- Mix together ¼ cup water and ¼ cup apple cider vinegar; rub mixture into your pet's skin every day for about a week, then weekly to control fleas.
- Run 1 cup apple cider vinegar or white vinegar in your empty dishwasher or empty washing machine monthly to clean out hard water buildup and to help remove odors.
- Clean gold jewelry by putting jewelry in a bowl and cover with apple cider vinegar or white vinegar for about 5 to 15 minutes; rinse and lightly brush with toothbrush if needed.

BENTONITE CLAY

Bentonite clay is decomposition of volcanic ash. I use other kinds of clay but my favorite clay to take internally is *Redmond Clay* from Utah. There are suggestions for internal & external uses throughout book.

Contains
Contains calcium, iron, magnesium, potassium, silica, sulphur and trace minerals (what minerals and nutrients the clay contains depend on where it comes from).

Internal Benefits
- Has antiviral, antifungal, antibacterial and disinfectant properties.
- Helps with digestion, gas, bloating, constipation, diarrhea, food poisoning, IBS, heartburn and acid reflux.
- Strengthens immune system and helps prevent bone loss.
- Reduces inflammation to help with arthritis issues and known to alleviate pain.
- Cleans the intestinal lining so we can absorb minerals and nutrients more efficiently. We absorb the nutrients that are present in the clay as well.

- Bentonite clay has a negative electromagnetic charge and most toxins have a positive charge to help remove toxins such as heavy metals, poisons, yeast and allergens from the body. Could also absorb some supplements and medications, so you should take clay at least 30 to 60 minutes before or after taking supplements or medications.

How to Take Bentonite Clay Internally
- **Bentonite clay water** - makes an alkaline mineral water. How to make - 1 teaspoon to 1 tablespoon of clay in a glass of any filtered water or distilled water (8 to 16 ounces), stir and let settle for 4 hours to overnight. The clay will collect at bottom of the glass. Drink the cloudy to clear water on top and leave the clay in bottom of glass. Drink 1 glass of clay water 1 to 3 times a day, preferably on an empty stomach. When it comes to relieving pain it may take a few days for clay to get into body's system and works best when taken daily.

Add 1 teaspoon to 1 tablespoon of clay to:
- Glass of water, juice or coconut water; stir and drink.
- Foods like applesauce, yogurt, pudding and oatmeal; stir and eat.
- Pet's water or food for nutrition and helps against fleas, worms or parasites.

FINGERNAIL IRREGULARITY MEANINGS

Fingernail beds should be colorless or light pink with a small white moon. These are some fingernail irregularities that can be related to diseases and health issues.

- Black nails or black spots can be a blood clot, heavy metals, fungal infection or cancer.
- Blue nails might not be getting enough oxygen, could indicate infection in lungs or pneumonia.
- Cracked or split nails can be a sign of iron deficiency, thyroid or kidney issues.
- Horizontal ridges or beau lines could be general malnutrition, blood sugar imbalance, fungal infection or side effect of chemotherapy.
- Nail bending or clubbing might mean that blood is not circulating properly, arthritis, heart, lung or liver issues.
- No moons can be underactive thyroid.
- Overly large moons can be overactive thyroid.
- Reddish, brownish streaks that look like splinters could be blood clots, heart issues or side effect of chemotherapy.
- Red nails can be heart, brain or lung issues.
- Spoon nails are nails that look scooped out which can be a sign of iron deficiency, anemia or thyroid issues.
- Unusual thick nails might mean that blood is not circulating properly.
- Unusual wide square nails can indicate hormonal imbalance.
- Vertical ridges can mean liver or stomach issues.
- White or pale nails can be anemia, liver issues or poisoning.
- White spots on nails could mean lacking minerals, malnutrition, blood sugar imbalance or arthritis.
- Yellow nails can be a fungal infection, blood sugar imbalance, and lung or thyroid issues

FOOT REFLEXOLOGY

An ancient method of massaging acupressure points in the feet that correspond to organs and other parts of the body. This bodywork involves application of massage and pressure to these points to stimulate body organs and relieve areas of congestion. Reflexology works with the body's energy flow (Qi or chi) along the meridians. Historically, reflexology is known to reduce pain, increase relaxation, stimulate circulation of blood and lymphatic fluids and much more. Best to use a reflexology practitioner or can do acupressure massage on your own feet. Foot reflexology is also used as a tool to find those sore spots on your feet to determine what organs or body areas may have health issues by using a foot reflexology chart. Knowing health issues we might have can be used as a tool to know what herbs and supplements to take. Another option is foot zoning.

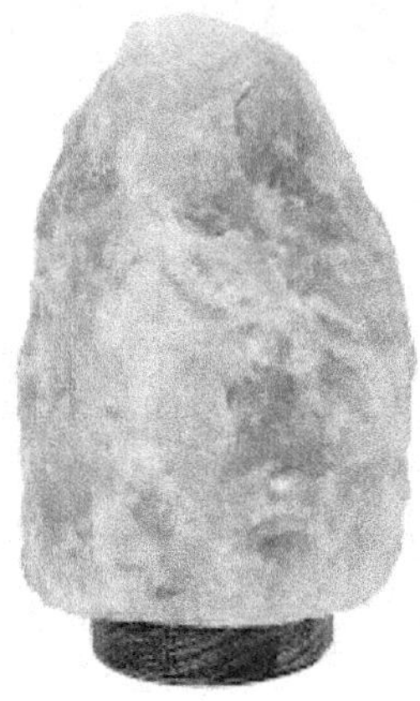

HIMALAYAN SEA SALT & SOLE WATER

True Himalayan sea salt comes from the Himalayan Mountains of Pakistan and is pink in color. It is known to contain the same 84 minerals including calcium, iron, magnesium, potassium, sodium and trace elements found in the human body. I use other sea salts but Himalayan sea salt is my favorite. There are suggestions for internal & external uses throughout book.

Himalayan salt lamps produce negative ions or invisible molecules which we inhale similar to those nature produces like being in the mountains, near waterfalls or at the beach and works as a natural ionizer to cleanse the air. They produce positive biochemical reactions that increase serotonin levels to help alleviate depression and stress. Salt lamps are known to improve sleep, help give a sense of well-being, neutralize the effects of electrical devices and cleanse negative energy.

Himalayan Sea Salt Internal Benefits
- Has antifungal, anti-bacterial and anti-inflammatory properties.
- Strengthens immune system.
- Decreases inflammation and pain.
- Your body will absorb minerals from salt when ingested or taking a bath.
- Helps harmonize the pH alkaline balance.
- Aids in maintaining healthier blood sugar and cholesterol levels.

How to Take Internally
- Buy fine Himalayan sea salt for using in home salt shakers or small sea salt pieces for salt grinder to use daily to season food and cooking.

- Add ½ teaspoon of Himalayan sea salt or sole water to glass of water or water bottle daily to absorb the minerals that the salt contains and to help promote a healthier balance of fluids and electrolytes.
- Make sole water.

Sole Water - Himalayan sea salt water

How to make sole water:
- Fill canning jar or glass jar with a lid ⅛ to ¼ full with any Himalayan sea salt pieces.
- Add spring water, purified water or distilled water, filling the container.
- After 24 hours salt should have dissolved and sole is ready to use.

External Himalayan Sea Salt Benefits & Uses
- Rub a smooth salt rock on under arms as a deodorant.
- Salt block to use for cooking.
- Himalayan sea salt necklaces are grounding and neutralize the effects of electrical devices and cleanse negative energy.
- Use the salt block healing room if your spa has one.

LEMON WATER

Lemon water is lemon juice squeezed from 1 to 2 lemons in a glass (8 ounces) of preferably room temperature to hot water.

Contains

Vitamins A, B6, C and calcium, copper, folate, hyaluronic acid, iron, magnesium, phosphorus, potassium, selenium and zinc.

Benefits of Drinking Lemon Water
- Has antiviral, antifungal and antibacterial properties.
- Increases hydration and helps harmonize the pH alkaline balance.
- Drink first thing in morning on an empty stomach to activate digestive system. Helps to liquefy and dump bile from liver and stimulate kidneys.
- Strengthens the immune system and is known to help dissolve kidney stones and gallstones.
- Assists the body in flushing toxins from the lymphatic system and dissolving uric acid.
- Is a natural antiseptic to help prevent bacteria from becoming an infection.
- Beneficial for throat issues, acid reflux, heartburn, bloating, constipation,

reduces phlegm, stomach and bladder issues.

Optional:
- To add lemon zest, grated ginger, raw honey or agave.
- Lemon ice cubes - juice big bag of lemons into an ice cube tray and freeze; add 1 to 3 cubes per glass of water.
- Make a pitcher of lemon water to drink throughout the day, using juice of 1 lemon per cup of water. Optional to add lemon ice cubes.

MASSAGE THERAPY

My thinking as a massage therapist is that a massage should help you heal and not just relax you. I prefer to give a therapeutic massage. I will use acupressure, reflexology, essential oils, stones, crystals, reiki, homemade healing herbal oils or salves, cranial work and energy work. While giving a massage, the body will indicate health concerns if you pay attention. For example, when clients have low back pain, under the eyes are puffy, ankles are swollen, need to urinate during massage and arch of feet are tender, these are symptoms that could indicate that their kidneys need some attention.

Health Benefits of Massage Therapy
- **Circulation** - improves oxygen supply and nutrients to cells and organs. Benefits glandular function, heart function and increases lymph circulation. Releases endorphins, which are hormones that act as our body's natural painkillers.
- **Muscular System** - loosens muscles and connective tissue. Helps reduce muscle spasms, cramping, soreness, stiffness, anxiety and tension. Also reduces post-surgery adhesions and edema. Improves range of motion and joint flexibility.
- **Skin** - stimulates blood to nourish skin and promotes tissue regeneration. Helps reduces scar tissue and stretch marks.

Some Healing Massage Techniques
- **Rolfing** - this technique utilizes deep physical manipulation and movement to bring the body into vertical alignment.
- **Shiatsu** - deep, finger-pressure technique using the traditional acupuncture points of Asian healing. Works to unblock energy flows and restore balance to meridians and organs.

- **Thai Yoga Massage** - modality that combines several techniques such as acupressure, stretching, breathing, energy work, herbal compresses and aromatherapy.

When you can't get a massage, you can use these massage tools on yourself to help loosen up muscles. These are some of my favorite tools that have helped me:
- Acupressure Balls & Canes
- Electric Massage Chairs & Tools
- Foot Balls & Rollers
- Gua Sha Tools
- Hard & Soft Foam Rollers

MEDICAL MARIJUANA

Medical marijuana or cannabis is an herb with many therapeutic benefits, it is used many ways including smoking, vapor, oils, salves, creams, butters, tinctures, extracts and edibles such as gummies, brownies, chocolates and much more. The cannabinoids in the herb bond with the receptors in the nerves and muscles, which is known to help relieve pain, headaches and reduce inflammation. Medical marijuana has a calming effect which helps muscles relax, improves sleep, reduces stress, anxiety and seizures. Has been known to help balance hormones and mood swings. Is known to increase appetite, boost creativity, prevent plaque buildup in the brain and reduce tumors. The cannabinoids also help control bacteria in the gut which helps aid digestion.

MEDITATION

Is a time-honored method for calming the mind and tuning in to your higher self. There are many studies indicating that the benefits of meditation may include stress relief, lower blood pressure, better sleep, anxiety reduction, increased breathing capacity and much more. Take time each day to sit quietly, breathe and release your thoughts to help you stay present to your life. So often we are thinking ahead or replaying the past and missing the gift of now. The present is where all the action is! Regular practice will positively impact your mind, body and spirit.

MINERALS & VITAMINS
NATURAL SOURCES

Calcium

A mineral that helps growth and maintenance of strong teeth, bone health, nervous system and muscle flexibility. Beneficial for healthier blood sugar levels, heart and lung health.

Foods - almond, aloe vera juice or gel, apricot, arugula, beas, blackstrap molasses, bok choy, bone broths, broccoli, cabbage, cheeses, chia seeds, collard green, cow's milk, dandelion green, date, fig, goji berry, goat's milk, kale, kefir, kiwi, lentils, maple syrup, mustard green, orange, peas, prickly pear, quinoa, rhubarb, royal jelly, salmon, sardine, seeds, soybean, tofu, turnip green, watercress and yogurts.

Herbs - alfalfa grass, barley grass, basil, borage, blue cohosh, blue violet, burdock, catnip, chamomile, chickweed, chicory, cilantro, cinnamon, coltsfoot, cramp bark, curry, damiana, dandelion, ecklonia cava, epazote, eyebright, goldenseal, green stevia, hops, horsetail, Irish moss, kelp, licorice root, maca, marjoram, mints, moringa, mullein, nettle, nutmeg, oat grass, oregano, paprika, parsley, peppermint, plantain, sage, red clover, red raspberry, rose hips, rosemary, sage, sarsaparilla, shepherd's purse, slippery elm, tamarind, thyme, turmeric, violet, leaf, watercress, wheatgrass, white oak bark, yarrow and yellow dock.

Chromium

It's the key to carbohydrate metabolism. Helps maintain healthier blood sugar, blood pressure and cholesterol levels.

Foods - apple, artichoke, asparagus, avocado, banana, barley, beans, beef, blackstrap molasses, broccoli, brewers' or nutritional yeast, broccoli, dates, eggs, garlic, grape juice, green bean, lettuces, mushrooms, oats, onion, oyster, nuts, pear, peas, peppers, potato, prune, strawberry, sweet potato, tomato, turkey, whole grains and cereals.

Herbs - basil, bilberry, black pepper, catnip, dulse, green tea, horsetail, juniper berry, licorice root, nettle, oat grass, red clover, sarsaparilla, thyme, wild yam and yarrow.

Copper

A mineral that helps in the formation of red blood cells and connective tissue. Is needed to produce collagen, a protein found in bones, ligaments, tendons, muscles, hair and nails. Beneficial for bone, heart and thyroid health.

Foods - acai berry, almond, aloe vera juice or gel, asparagus, avocado, beef, blackstrap molasses, 100% cacao or raw cacao nibs, cashew, chia seeds, collard green, crab, eggs, flaxseeds, garbanzo bean, hazelnut, kale, kiwi, lentils, livers, lobster, mushrooms, mustard green, oyster, peas, quinoa, radish, royal jelly, sardine, scallion, sesame seed, soybean, spinach, sun dried tomato, sunflower seed, swiss chard, tuna, turnip green and walnut.

Herbs - alfalfa grass, bilberry, burdock, celery seed, chamomile, chickweed, cumin, echinacea, horsetail, kelp, maca, marshmallow root, nutmeg, parsley, pine pollen, red clover, red raspberry, rosemary, sheep sorrel, slippery elm, thyme, wheatgrass and yarrow.

Other Source - copper infused water: store water for 8 hours to overnight in 100% copper vessel, for instance a pitcher, mug or water bottle, drink 1 to 2 glasses a day.

Folate

Folate or vitamin B9 helps form healthier red blood cells. Helps with anemia, as well as repairs and stimulates healthier cell growth. Beneficial for brain, colon and heart health.

Foods - almond, asparagus, arugula, avocado, banana, beans, beef, bee pollen, beet & green, broccoli, brown rice, brussel sprout, cabbage, cantaloupe, cauliflower, citrus fruits, collard green, dandelion green, egg yolk, hazelnut, kale, kiwi, lentils, legumes, mushrooms, okra, papaya, peas, quinoa, romaine lettuce, rhubarb, royal jelly, spinach, turnip green and wheat germ.

Herbs - alfalfa grass, barley grass, basil, burdock, chamomile, chlorella, cilantro, epazote, hawthorn berry, oat grass, oregano, parsley, pine pollen, red raspberry, rosemary, sage, thyme, wheatgrass and yellow dock.

Iodine

A mineral that helps maintain healthy thyroid function. Benefits bone and brain health, improves hair growth and protects against radiation.

Foods - sea vegetables contain the most, including alaria, arame, bladder wrack, dulse, chlorella, Irish moss, hijiki, kelp, kombu, krill oil, nori, spirulina & wakame (can eat, powder form or supplement products). Followed by asparagus, cabbage, cheddar cheese, cod, cod liver oil, cow's milk, eggs, fish bone broths, goat's milk, haddock, lobster, mushrooms, peas, potato, salmon, sardine, scallop, sea bass, shrimp, swiss chard, tuna, turkey breast, turnip green, watercress and yogurt.

Herbs - black pepper, black walnut, bugleweed, dandelion, ecklonia cava, fennel, hyssop, lemon balm, motherwort, sarsaparilla, tarragon leaf and turkey rhubarb.

Iron

A mineral that helps fight against anemia and benefits muscles and brain health. If you have dark circles under your eyes and are tired all the time, these maybe a sign that you are low on iron. Pull down bottom eyelid to see if pale. If there are lots of red blood vessels, then iron is good.

Foods - egg yolk, red meats & liver probably contain the most. Followed by apricot kernel, beans, beet & green, blackstrap molasses, bone broths, broccoli, 100% cacao or raw cacao nibs, chia seeds, chicken, collard green, dandelion green, fig, flaxseeds, green bean, kale, lentils, lettuces, maple syrup, natto, nuts, oyster, peach, pear, peas, pecan, pork, prune, quinoa, raisin, royal jelly, sardine, scallop, seeds, spinach, sprouts, strawberry, tofu, turkey and watermelon.

Herbs - alfalfa grass, anise, barley grass, basil, barberry, bilberry, bladderwrack, blue cohosh, blue violet, burdock, catnip, cayenne, chamomile, chickweed, chicory, cilantro, clove, comfrey, curry, dandelion, dong quai, dulse, echinacea, ecklonia cava, eyebright, fennel, fenugreek, ginger, goldenseal, green stevia, hibiscus, horehound, kelp, lemongrass, licorice root, maca, milk thistle, marshmallow root, mints, moringa, mullein, nettle, nutmeg, oat grass, oregano, paprika, parsley, pine pollen, plantain, red raspberry leaf, red clover, rosemary, sarsaparilla, skullcap, sheep sorrel, shepherd's purse, slippery elm, suma, tamarind, turmeric, thyme, uva ursi, wheatgrass, white oak bark, yarrow, yellow dock and yerba mate.

Other Sources - yellow dock root decoction (see Herbs/Tea)

Magnesium

A mineral that is needed to prevent calcification of soft tissue and promotes healthy bones. Magnesium helps to keep the nerves relaxed, reduces inflammation and helps against muscular twitching. Assists in mineral absorption and is known as nature's laxative. Helps maintain healthier blood sugar and cholesterol levels.

Foods - acai berry, almond, aloe vera juice or gel, apple, arugula, avocado, banana, barley, beet & green, beans, blackstrap molasses, bone broths, broccoli, brown rice, brussel sprout, buckwheat, 100% cacao or raw cacao nibs, chia seeds, collard green, dandelion green, flaxseeds, garlic, ginger, guava, lentils, lettuces, maple syrup, millet, noni juice, nuts, oats, okra, onion, oyster, peas, prickly pear cactus, quinoa, salmon, sardine, seeds, spinach, sprouts, swiss chard, tofu and wheat germ.

Herbs - alfalfa grass, barley grass, basil, bladderwrack, black cohosh, burdock, catnip, cayenne, celery seed, chamomile, chervil, chickweed, cilantro, clove, coriander, curry, dandelion, dulse, ecklonia cava, eyebright, fennel, fenugreek, ginger, green stevia, green tea, gotu kola, hops, horsetail, jackfruit, juniper berry, kelp, lemongrass, licorice root, maca, mullein, nettle, nutmeg, oat grass, oregano, paprika, parsley, pine pollen, sage, red clover, red raspberry, red clover, rosehips, rosemary, saffron, sage, sheep sorrel, shepherd's purse, slippery elm, tarragon, valerian, watercress, wheatgrass, willow, wood betony, yarrow and yellow dock.

Potassium

A mineral which helps the development of bones, teeth, nerves and strengthen muscles. Helps maintain electrolyte and fluid balance to help balance pH in the body. Beneficial for kidney and heart health.

Foods - acai berry, acorn squash, aloe vera juice or gel, apple, apricot, arugula, avocado, asparagus, banana & stem, beans, beet & greens, bitter melon, bone broths, broccoli, brussel sprout, cabbage, cantaloupe, cauliflower, carrot, carrot juice, celery, cherry, chia seeds, clam, cucumber, dandelion green, date, edamame, elderberry, fig, flaxseeds, ginger, goji berry, green bean, kefir, kiwi, lemon, lime, maple syrup, mushrooms, mustard green, orange, peas, pineapple, prickly pear cactus, prune, quinoa, radish, raison, royal jelly, salmon, seeds, spinach, sweet potato, swiss chard, tomato sauce, turnip green, watermelon, winter squash, yams and yogurts.

Herbs - alcachofa, alfalfa grass, barley grass, birch, black & blue cohosh, borage, blue violet, burdock, catnip, cayenne, chamomile, chaparral, chicory, cilantro, clove, coltsfoot, comfrey, dandelion, dill, dulse, echinacea, ecklonia cava, epazote, eyebright, fennel, ginger, grape, hops, horsetail, juniper berry, kelp, licorice root, maca, mullein, nettle, nutmeg, oat grass, oregano, papaya, parsley, peppermint, pine pollen, plantain, red clover, red raspberry, rosehips, rosemary, saffron, skullcap, slippery elm, tamarind, thyme, turmeric, wheatgrass, wintergreen and yarrow.

Selenium

A mineral that benefits hormone, prostate and thyroid health. Strengthens immune system and aids with muscles, eyes and teeth health.

Foods - avocado, asparagus, banana, beef, blackstrap molasses, blueberry, bone broths, brewers' or nutritional yeast, broccoli, brown rice, cabbage, coconut, collard green, cheeses, chicken, crab, date, eggs, flaxseeds, goji berry, gooseberry, liver, lobster, mushrooms, mussel, nuts, oats, oyster, peach, pineapple, pomegranate seed, pork, raisin, rye bread, salmon, sardine, scallop, seeds, shrimp, snapper, spinach, strawberry, tuna and turkey.

Herbs - alfalfa grass, buckthorn, burdock, catnip, cayenne, chamomile, chaparral, chickweed, comfrey, dulse, epazote, fennel, fenugreek, green stevia, hawthorn berry, horsetail, juniper berry, kelp, lemongrass, lobelia, marshmallow root, milk thistle, nettle, nutmeg, oat grass, parsley, peppermint, pine pollen, red raspberry, red clover, rosehips, sarsaparilla, slippery elm, uva ursi, wheatgrass, yarrow and yellow dock.

Silica

A mineral to help strengthen and repair bones, tendons, muscles, connective tissues and cartilage. Helps with maintaining healthier nervous system, teeth, nails, skin and hair. Beneficial for lungs, kidney, bladder and brain health.

Foods - apple, asparagus, banana, barley, beet, bell pepper, bone broths, brown rice, cabbage, carrot, celery, corn, cucumber, fig, flaxseeds, garbanzo bean, garlic, grape, green bean, kale, lettuces, leek, lentils, mango, millet, oats, onion, potato, radish, raison, royal jelly, soybean, spinach, strawberry, tomato and watercress.

Herbs - horsetail probably contains the most. Followed by alfalfa grass, bamboo, burdock, kelp, marjoram, nettle, oat grass, parsley, rosehips and wheatgrass.

Other Sources - bentonite clay & food grade diatomaceous earth.

Zinc

A mineral known to improve mental alertness, strengthen immune system, reduces inflammation and assists in wound healing.

Foods - aloe vera juice or gel, arugula, asparagus, avocado, beef, beans, bone broths, 100% cacao or raw cacao nibs, cauliflower, chia seeds, chicken, collard green, cow's milk, crab, flaxseeds, garlic, goat's milk, horseradish, lamb, lentils, lobster, mango, maple syrup, mushrooms, nuts, oats, okra, oyster, quinoa, seeds, shrimp, soybean, spinach, turkey and wheat germ.

Herbs - acerola, alfalfa grass, barberry, bilberry, burdock, cayenne, chamomile, chickweed, coltsfoot, dandelion, epazote, eyebright, fennel, ginger, hops, horehound, horsetail, juniper berry, kelp, licorice root, maca, marshmallow root, milk thistle, mints, mullein, nettle, parsley, red clover, rosehips, rosemary, sage, sarsaparilla, sheep sorrel, skullcap, slippery elm, thyme, wheatgrass and wild yam.

Vitamin A

Helps benefit eye health, strengthen immune system and beneficial for bone and cell growth. Helps keep eyes, skin and mucous membranes moist.

Foods - acai berry, apricot kernel, artichoke, arugula, banana, beet & green, bone broths, brewers' or nutritional yeast, brussel sprout, cabbage, cantaloupe, carrot, celery, cheeses, cherry, clam, cod liver oil, collard green, whole cow's milk, dandelion green, eggs, elderberry, fish oils, garlic, goat's milk, goji berry, golden berry, kale, mango, mustard green, nuts, oyster, papaya, peach, peas, prune, pineapple, pomegranate seed, pumpkin seed, red palm oil, royal jelly, sacha inchi seed, salmon, shark liver oil, spinach, star fruit, sweet potato, swiss chard, tomato, trout, tuna, turnip greens, watermelon and yacon root.

Herbs - acerola, alfalfa grass, basil, bilberry, blue violet, borage, burdock, catnip, cayenne, chamomile, chaparral, chickweed, cilantro, clove, comfrey, curry leaf, dandelion, ecklonia cava, epazote, eyebright, flaxseeds, ginger, goldenseal, hibiscus, hops, horsetail, kelp, lemongrass, licorice root, marjoram, marshmallow root, milk thistle, mullein, nettle, noni and juice, nutmeg, oat grass, oregano, paprika, parsley, peppermint, persimmon, plantain, pine pollen, red clover, red raspberry, rosehips, rosemary, safflower, saffron, sage, uva ursi, thyme, wheatgrass and yellow dock.

Vitamin B12

B12 or cobalamin is needed to produce enough healthier red blood cells in the bone marrow and to properly metabolize food to produce energy. It helps to prevent anemia, aids digestive system, brain health and helps to form myelin.

Foods - almond, asparagus, bee pollen, beef, brewers' or nutritional yeast, 100%

cacao or raw cacao nibs, cheeses, chicken, clam, crab, whole cow's milk, eggs, goat's milk, goji berry, kale, kefir, kidney, lamb, liver, lobster, mackerel, miso, mushrooms, mustard green, lobster, mussel, okra, oyster, poultry, royal jelly, salmon, sardine, scallop, shrimp, spinach, swiss chard, tofu, tuna, turkey and yogurt.

Herbs - alfalfa grass, barberry, barley grass, bladderwrack, burdock, catnip, chamomile, chickweed, dandelion, dong quai, dulse, fenugreek, forskohlii, lecithin, hawthorn berry, hops, kelp, maca, milk thistle, nettle, oat grass, red raspberry, safflower, sage, wheatgrass, white oak bark and yellow dock.

Vitamin B17

B17 or amygdalin is known to reduce tumors, helps to control blood pressure and strengthen immune system.

Foods - apricot kernel or seeds probably have the most. Followed by bamboo shoot, barley, beet & green, bitter almond, blackberry, black radish, blueberry, brown rice, garbanzo bean, cherry seed, cranberry, elderberry, fava bean, flaxseeds, garbanzo bean, gooseberry, kidney bean, lentils, macadamia, millet, mung bean, peach seed, pear seed, plum seed, prune seed, raspberry, royal jelly, sprouts, strawberry, squash and sweet potato.

Herbs - alfalfa grass, bamboo, eucalyptus, lecithin, nettle and watercress.

Vitamin C

Is a wound healer, stimulates growth and repair of tissues in your body. Helps calcium and iron formation and strengthens immune system.

Foods - acai berry, aloe vera juice or gel, amalaki fruit, apple, arugula, asparagus, avocado, banana, bee pollen, bitter melon, blackberry, blackcurrant, black radish, blueberry, brazil nut, broccoli, brussel sprout, cabbage, cauliflower, cherry, cantaloupe, collard green, cucumber, dragon fruit, elderberry, garlic, green bean, goji berry, gooseberry, grapefruit, green bean, guava, horseradish, jackfruit, juniper berry, kale, kiwi, lemon, lemongrass, lime, lychee, mango, maple syrup, melons, mustard green, orange, okra, onion, papaya, peach, peas, peppers, persimmon, pineapple, pomegranate seed, pomelo, potato, prune, pumpkin, radish, raspberry, royal jelly, scallion, spinach, squash, star fruit, strawberry, sunchoke, sweet potato, swiss chard, tangerine, tomato, turnip green, watercress, watermelon, yacon root and zucchini.

Herbs - acerola, amla berry, camu camu & rosehips probably contain the most.

Followed by alcachofa, alfalfa grass, barberry, barley grass, barberry, basil, bilberry, blue violet, burdock, boneset, catnip, cayenne, chamomile, chickweed, chives, cilantro, cloves, coltsfoot, curry, dandelion, eyebright, fennel, green stevia, green tea, hawthorn berry, hibiscus, hops, horsetail, kelp, licorice root, lobelia, maca, marshmallow root, milk thistle, moringa, mullein, nettle, nutmeg, oat grass, oregano, paprika, parsley, peppermint, plantain, papaya, red clover, red raspberry, rosemary, saffron, skullcap, slippery elm, tamarind, turmeric, thyme, violet leaf, wheatgrass, yarrow and yellow dock.

Vitamin D

Is known to help regulate body's bone development, cell growth and strengthen immune system. Beneficial for bones, teeth, lungs, thyroid and brain health.

Foods - cod liver oil contains the most. Followed by almond milk, bee pollen, beef, catfish, caviar, cheeses, cow's milk, eggs, eel, fish oils, flaxseeds, goat's milk, herring, kefir, lettuces, livers, mackerel, mushrooms, oats, oyster, pork, royal jelly, salmon, sardine, shrimp, soy milk, tofu, trout, tuna and yogurts.

Herbs - alfalfa grass, chickweed, dandelion, eyebright, fenugreek, horsetail, lemongrass, mullein, nettle, parsley and watercress.

Other Sources - sunlight 15 minutes on both sides of body daily without using sunscreen.

Vitamin E

Helps strengthen immune system, repair tissue, produce red blood cells, improves circulation and promotes healthier skin and hair.

Foods - aloe vera juice or gel, apricot kernel, asparagus, avocado, bee pollen, bell pepper, broccoli, 100% cacao or raw cacao nibs, chia seeds, coconut oil, collard green, eggs, evening primrose oil, flaxseeds, herring, kiwi, mango, mustard green, nuts, olive oil, papaya, pomegranate seed, pumpkin seed, quinoa, red palm oil, royal jelly, sacha inchi seed & oil, safflower seed & oil, salmon, sesame seed & oil, spinach, squash, sunflower seed & oil, sweet potato, swordfish, swiss chard, swordfish, tomato, trout, turnip green, wheat germ and yacon root.

Herbs - acerola, alfalfa grass, barley grass, bilberry, cayenne, cilantro, cinnamon, dandelion, dong quai, ginger, green tea, goldenseal, kelp, maca, milk thistle, neem, nettle, oat grass, oregano, red clover, red raspberry, rosehips, sage, tamarind, thyme, watercress and wheatgrass.

Vitamin K

Helps the blood in our bodies to coagulate. Needed to form and repair bones and injuries. Beneficial for brain and digestive health.

Foods - arugula, asparagus, avocado, bee pollen, beet green, blackberry, blueberry, broccoli, brussel sprout, cabbage, cauliflower, collard green, dandelion green, egg yolk, endive, green bean, kale, kefir, mustard green, natto powder, okra, olive oil, pomegranate seed, prune, pumpkin seed, romaine lettuce, spinach, swiss chard, turnip green and wheat germ.

Herbs - alfalfa grass, basil, bilberry, cayenne, cilantro, clove, coriander, green tea, kelp, marjoram, nettle, oat grass, oregano, parsley, plantain, red raspberry, sage, shepherd's purse, thyme and wheatgrass.

Some Natural Sources to Get Minerals & Vitamins
- Apple cider vinegar.
- Bentonite clay.
- Bone broths.
- Coral calcium supplements.Goat whey protein powder.
- Hemp hearts.
- Hemp protein powder.
- Himalayan sea salt & sole water.
- Liquid chlorophyll.
- Oyster shell supplements.
- Powdered greens.
- Sea vegetables such as alaria, arame, bladderwrack, chlorella, nori, dulse, ecklonia cava, Irish moss, kelp, kombu, spirulina & wakame. (can eat, powder form or supplement products).
- Whey protein powder.

POWDERED GREENS

Powdered greens are a whole food source, a multi nutritional supplement combination. Best to buy a powdered greens supplement made without sugars or unnatural fillers. Or you can make your own combination.

Benefits of Powdered Greens
- Is a whole food and herbal nutritional supplement containing high amounts of minerals, vitamins, fiber, digestive enzymes and protein.
- Increases natural energy, stamina and strengthens immune system.
- Helps harmonize the pH alkaline balance.
- Helps reduce inflammation and stimulates growth of new tissue.
- Aids in maintaining healthier blood sugar, blood pressure and cholesterol levels.
- Is known to improve mental clarity and focus.
- Helps detoxify toxins such as heavy metals from the body.

Some Ingredient Suggestions for Making Powdered Greens Combination
- Alfalfa Grass Powder
- Amla Berry Powder
- Apple Pectin Powder
- Asparagus Powder
- Barley Grass Powder
- Beet Root Powder
- Blue Violet Powder
- Broccoli Powder
- Camu Camu Powder
- Carrot Powder
- Chaga Mushroom Powder
- Chlorella Powder
- Cucumber Seed Powder
- Dandelion Powder
- Ginger Powder
- Green Stevia Powder
- Green Tea Powder
- Kelp Powder
- Moringa Powder
- Myrrh Powder
- Nettle Powder
- Oat Grass Powder
- Parsley Powder
- Peppermint Powder
- Reishi Mushroom Powder
- Red Raspberry Powder
- Royal Jelly Powder
- Rosehip Powder
- Spirulina Powder
- Spinach Powder
- Wheatgrass Powder
- Yellow Dock Powder

Sample Powdered Greens Recipe
- 5 ounces Alfalfa Grass powder
- 5 ounces Barley Grass Powder
- 3 ounces Oat Grass Powder
- 3 ounces Wheatgrass Powder
- 2 ounces Nettle Powder
- 2 ounces Green Stevia Powder
- 1 ounce Dandelion Powder
- 1 ounce Amla Berry Powder

- 2 ounce Moringa Powder   • 1 ounce Peppermint Powder

Mix ingredients together and store in closed containers.

How to Take Powdered Greens
- Basic recipe: mix 1 teaspoon to 1 tablespoon of powder 1 or 2 times daily with a liquid such as water, juice, coconut water, herbal tea or almond milk; stir and drink.
- Add 1 teaspoon to 1 tablespoon to applesauce, yogurt, pudding, oatmeal, protein powder blender drink or whole food blender drink.
- Make a tincture or encapsulate the powder. You will need to take 3 to 9 squirts of tincture or about 4 to 12 capsules a day to equal 1 teaspoon to 1 tablespoon of powder.
- Add ¼ to 1 teaspoon to pet's water and/or food or in watering can for plants and garden.

REIKI (pronounced ray-key)

Discovered in 1922 by Dr. Mikao Usui, a Buddhist Christian schoolmaster in Japan. Reiki is not associated with any religion. It is a light touch healing technique which gently facilitates each person's own ability to find and maintain balance in the body, mind and spirit. The reiki practitioner uses visualization and acts as a channel for the life force energy (Qi or Chi). This energy is transferred from one person to another through the hands of a Reiki practitioner by holding the hands on or above the parts of the body that requires healing. Every part of the body receives treatment as the Reiki energy travels through the entire body, although it is concentrated on the spot where the hands are held. Some benefits are headache relief, improved sleep, reducing aches and pains, better digestion, strengthen immune system and much more.

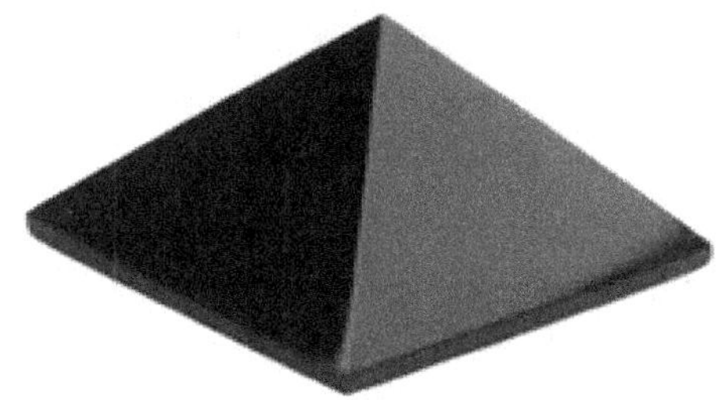

STONES & CRYSTALS

Each type of stone or crystal gives off their own unique form of subtle energy. They resonate with the different energies in each person to benefit your physical and mental well-being. There are suggestions for uses throughout book.

Some of the Various Benefits Associated With the Following Stones & Crystals

- **Amber** - calming, eyesight, clarity, purifies the spirit and throat issues.
- **Amethyst** - intuition, dreams, healing, peace, love, grief, prosperity, promotes sobriety, protection, travel, wisdom, opens psychic center and headaches.
- **Aquamarine** - promotes courage, purification, balance, intuition, protection and protects against gossip.
- **Aventurine** - healing, money, motivation, leadership and luck.
- **Black Obsidian** - very grounding, protection, help clear negative thoughts and release old patterns.
- **Black Onyx** - guards against negativity, promotes self-confidence and courage, helps heal emotional wounds and strength to start new.
- **Black Tourmaline** - strong grounding stone, helps you face difficult situations, calms panic attacks and promotes self-confidence.
- **Carnelian** - concentration, assertiveness, awareness, self-esteem, action, grief, protection from bad vibes and calms temper.
- **Citrine** - wealth, attracts money, protection, intuition, comfort, self-esteem, digestion, depression, gives joy, confidence and energy.
- **Garnet** - removes negativity, insight, health and promotes physical healing.
- **Hematite** - grounding, improved concentration, focus, sleep and blocks negativity energy.

- **Jade** - good luck, protection, longevity, healing properties, attracts true love, releases negative thoughts and promotes good dreams.
- **Jasper** - grounding, stress, calming, replenish energy, promotes courage and confidence.
- **Lapis** - self-confidence, friendship, intuition, creativity and clears throat for speaking up.
- **Malachite** - peaceful sleep, emotions, speeds healing, travel, clears blocked energy, helpful against radiation, tumors, helps with pain and circulation.
- **Moonstone** - relationships, harmony, attraction, good fortune and intuition.
- **Quartz Crystal** - universal stone, enhance ability to enjoy life, stimulates brain function and strengthen inner healing abilities.
- **Rose Quartz** - love stone, sense of self-worth, grief, open heart to love and gives inner peace.
- **Smoky Quartz** - protects against negativity, grounding, improves focus, relaxing, depression, reduces stress and travel.
- **Sodalite** - meditation, healing, harmony and understanding.
- **Tiger's eye** - protection attracts money, leadership, strength and past life understanding.
- **Turquoise** - good luck, symbol of wealth, healing stone, strengthen immune system and protects against negative energy.

Carry stones & crystals with you in your pocket, purse, bra, watch, or as jewelry. The type of stone or crystal you select depends on what benefits you seek, such as amethyst geode to eliminate negative energy from home or workplace. Maybe put a piece of citrine in your wallet or cash register to attract money. Wear smoky quartz when you are around negative people or rose quartz to attract love.

Clean & clear any negative energy from the stones or crystals & re-energize them by using one or all these techniques:
- Bury in bowl of sea salt
- Rinse in a waterfall or under running water
- Place outside in the moonlight

WATER & HYDRATION

Hydration plays a much more major role in our health than most people imagine. Water comprises 60 to 80% of our bodies. Without replenishing water, the body simply cannot function at a basic healthy level. Any unsweetened plain water will do, but probably better to drink filtered, purified, spring or distilled water.

Signs You May Be Dehydrated
- Feeling thirsty.
- Bags under eyes.
- Deep vertical lines on lips.
- Headaches, dizziness, fatigue, brain fog and/or lightheadedness.
- Dry skin, mouth, tongue, hair, eyes and/or nose.
- Hemorrhoids, constipation and/or small hard feces.
- Irregular body temperatures.
- Skin can feel cool and clammy.
- Colon and digestive problems.
- Tightness and/or cramps in muscles and joints.
- Urine is dark yellow, smelly and/or infrequent. Urine should be clear to pale yellow and not very smelly.

Ways to Get More Hydrated
- Drink plenty of unsweetened plain water, at least half your body weight in ounces daily. For example; if you weigh 200 pounds, then you should keep increasing water intake to get to 100 ounces of water or six 16 ounce water bottles daily.
- Drink whole food blender drink - consider including some of the foods listed below.
- Make infused water by adding produce or herbs like slices of lemon, lime, cucumber, all berries, pomegranate seeds, pineapple, cherry, watermelon, hibiscus, fresh mint or basil leaf into a pitcher of water, canning jar infuser or bottles with a grinder on bottom.
- 1 to 3 tablespoons of chia gel.
- Eat and incorporate healthy oils. Take 1 to 3 tablespoons a day such as extra virgin olive oil, grapeseed oil, safflower oil or sesame oil.
- Eat produce that contain lots of water like apple, apricot, asparagus, banana, beet, blackberry, blueberry, broccoli, butterhead lettuce, cabbage, cantaloupe, carrot, cauliflower, cranberry, celery, cherry, cucumber, dragon fruit, eggplant, endive, grapefruit, grape, honeydew, iceberg

lettuce, kiwi, lemon, leek, lime, mango, mangosteen, mushrooms, onion, orange, papaya, peas, peach, pear, peppers, pineapple, plum, pomegranate seeds, radish, raspberry, rhubarb, romaine lettuce, spinach, star fruit, strawberry, swiss chard, tomato, watermelon and zucchini.
- Soak in warm bath water for about 15 to 45 minutes.

Also good to drink:
- Coconut water
- Unsweetened herbal tea - herb suggestions include alfalfa, chamomile, hibiscus, mints, nettle, red raspberry leaf or rosehip.
- Glass of water with pinch of sea salt or ½ teaspoon of sole water.
- Lemon Water (see Lemon Water).
- Sports/Electrolyte Drink (see DIY Recipes).

Miscellaneous Water Information
- A glass of water or cup of tea universally equals 8 ounces.
- Sometimes when people are dehydrated, they mistake thirst for hunger and can overeat trying to get water the body needs.
- Drinking 1 to 2 glasses of water before eating a meal can act as an appetite suppressant.
- Two glasses of water first thing in morning helps to activate our colon and internal organs.
- Any fluid while eating a meal can dilute the acid in the stomach resulting in slower digestion. Drinking fluids before or after a meal would be wiser.
- Cold water after a meal may not always be a good idea. Cold water passing through our system solidifies the oily foods just eaten and can possibly slow down digestion and elimination. Drink warm water, herbal tea or broth after a meal to prevent any oils solidifying.
- Slow down and give your body a chance to absorb the water you're drinking. Gulping water is counterproductive.

WHOLE FOOD BLENDER DRINKS

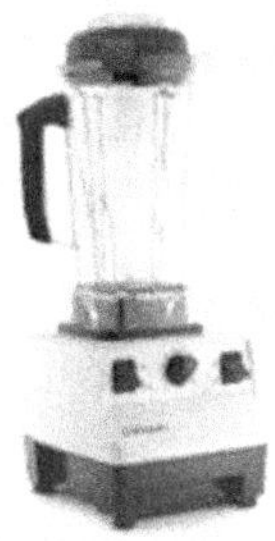

Many nutrients available in raw produce is held within the indigestible fiber or that part of the fruit and vegetables the body naturally expels. However, when fruit or vegetables are blended, these nutrients are released from the fiber and easily absorbed into the bloodstream. Blender drinks should be made from raw fruits and vegetables. If possible, use organic. Frozen, dried or dehydrated produce is the next best option.

Why Organic?

We are depleting our soils of nutrition. A cup of produce grown in the year 1900 contained 30 to 60 times more nutrition than our common fruits and vegetables grown today. We obtain much more nutrition from organic foods which are grown on environmentally and animal friendly farms using fertile soil by rotating crops and using compost and manure instead of artificial chemical fertilizers, pesticides or additives. Animals that are pasture raised, cage free or free range and not given steroids, antibiotics and artificial growth hormones are preferred. You should also consider organic dairy products, meats, poultry, eggs, baby food, baby products and so forth. If none of these options are available, do the best you can.

Juicing vs Blending

Juicing extracts fluid from produce and throws away the indigestible fiber. If you have a sensitive digestive system or illness that prevents your body from processing fiber, juicing might be a better choice for you.

Benefits of Whole Food Blender Drinks
- When you blend, most likely you will consume more fruits and vegetables than you would probably actually eat.
- Blending is an easy way to provide you with a high level of quality fiber and nutrition.
- Increases energy level and strengthens immune system.

- Fruits and vegetables in their raw state have high water content so whole food blender drinks aid better hydration.

Things to Consider Before You Blend
- Clean produce - soak produce in ¼ cup of white or apple cider vinegar in a ½ to full gallon of water for 5 minutes or more. Rinse to remove as much dirt and chemicals as you can.
- The skin of citrus fruits contain an oil that is not easily digested so best to cut off skin while leaving the pith on citrus.
- Adding ½ to 1 cup of ice or using frozen fruit can make your drink colder and may taste better to some people.

Whole Food Blender Drink Recipe Example
- ½ cup of spinach
- 2 kale leaves
- 1 carrot
- 1 celery stalk
- 1 small apple
- 2 to 3 prunes
- 1 tablespoon of chia seeds
- Few fresh parsley leaves
- ½ cup of ice
- 1 cup of distilled water

For Whole Food Blender Drinks
- Use 1 to 3 cups of liquid per drink suggested as the base. Liquid suggestions include filtered water, distilled water, juice, aloe vera juice, coconut water, coconut milk or almond milk.
- Feel free to just use whatever produce you have, but using 5 or more produce per drink works well.
- Each drink should be 8 to 20 ounces and try to drink 1 to 3 drinks per day.
- Suggestion - also blend hot vegetable soups.
- Experiment, create your own recipes and have fun!

Produce Suggestions for Blending

- Acai Berry or Juice
- Apple (remove stem)
- Apricot
- Arugula Green
- Asparagus
- Avocado & Avocado Seed
- Banana
- Beet & Leaf
- Bitter Melon
- Blackberry
- Blueberry
- Broccoli Tops & Stem
- Brussel Sprout
- Cabbage
- Carrot
- Cauliflower
- Celery & Celery Root
- Cherry (remove pit)
- Cinnamon Stick or Powder
- Coconut
- Collard Green
- Corn (cut off the cob)
- Cranberry
- Cucumber
- Dandelion Green
- Date
- Dragon Fruit
- Elderberry
- Endive Leaf
- Fig
- Ginger Root
- Goji Berry
- Grape
- Grapefruit
- Green Bean
- Green Onion
- Kale Leaf
- Kiwi
- Lemon
- Lime
- Mango
- Mangosteen Fruit & Juice
- Mushrooms
- Mustard Green
- Nectarine
- Noni Fruit & Juice
- Onion
- Orange
- Papaya
- Peach
- Peppers
- Persimmon
- Pineapple & Stem
- Pomegranate Seeds
- Prune
- Radish & Leaf
- Raspberry
- Spinach Leaf
- Sprouts
- Star Fruit
- Strawberry
- Swiss Chard Leaf
- Watercress Leaf
- Zucchini

Ingredients to Consider

- Apricot Kernel
- Cacao Powder or Raw Cacao
- Chia Seeds
- Chyawanprash
- Cooked Beans
- Flaxseed Meal
- Hemp Hearts
- Kefir
- Non-GMO Lecithin
- Liquid Chlorophyll
- Natto Powder
- Nuts
- Powdered Greens
- Protein Powders
- Raw Honey
- Royal Jelly
- Seeds
- Yogurt

Fresh Cut Herbs

- Basil Leaf
- Cilantro Leaf
- Curry Leaf
- Green Stevia Leaf
- Marijuana Leaf
- Mint Leaf
- Oat Grass
- Oregano Leaf
- Parsley Leaf
- Peppermint Leaf
- Rosemary Leaf
- Thyme Leaf

SUGGESTIONS FOR VARIOUS HEALTH ISSUES

BETTER BRAIN

The brain is the body's main control center. The brain controls the body's motor skills, emotions, rational thinking, obsessions, memory and way more. Part of the body's hormone endocrine glands are at the brain: the pineal gland, pituitary gland and hypothalamus gland.

General Symptoms that the Brain Needs Attention
- Headaches or migraines.
- Loss of memory or seizures.
- Hard to concentrate or hyperactive.
- Unbalanced posture, will bump into things.
- Nausea or vomiting.
- Sensitivity to light and sound.
- Change in behavior.
- Muscle twitching.
- Lack of muscle control.
- Speech or vision problems.
- Lactating when not pregnant.
- Alzheimer's, autism, and Parkinson's.

Natural Suggestions to Strengthen the Brain
- Get enough sleep - 6 to 9 hours nightly.
- Occasional day of fasting to help clean system of toxins.
- Relax - suggestions are slow down, listen to calming music, get plenty of sleep, do meditation, walk labyrinths and find some alone time.
- Acupuncture, chiropractic or massage therapy.
- Keep brain busy for instance reading, doing puzzles, playing games or taking a class.
- Switch to natural household and personal care products or make your own DIY products.
- Hyperbaric oxygen therapy.
- Stones & crystals - amber, amethyst, lapis, moonstone, sodalite or quartz. Carry with you or on you, as jewelry, in your pocket, in your purse or lie down with stones on forehead.

- Essential oils & reflexology to benefit the brain - basil, bergamot, geranium, helichrysum, lemon, myrrh, neroli, peppermint, rose, rosemary, sage or sandalwood. Choose your own blend and use in a spray, roll-on, eye pillow, diffuser, car diffuser, bath salts, body oil, massage oil or lotion. Mix 3 to 10 drops in 1 to 3 tablespoons any carrier oil & massage toes or scalp.

Internally
- Eat healthier & drink plenty of water.
- Whole food blender drink daily - ingredient suggestions are acai berry, avocado, beet, blueberry, cordycep, goji berry, kale, lecithin, pomegranate seed & juice, pumpkin seed, spinach, reishi mushroom and sage leaf.
- Eggs - best to look for pasture raised, cage free or free range; nutrients in eggs help regulate brain chemicals.
- Apple cider vinegar drink - 1 tablespoon each of apple cider vinegar and raw honey in glass of warm water; stir and drink 1 to 3 times a day.
- Bone broth, gelatin or collagen powder - best to look for grass-fed, pasture raised or organic.
- Bone broths including beef, chicken, fish, lamb or turkey.
- Omega fatty acids.
- Mushroom supplement products or tea.
- Non-GMO lecithin products.
- Sea vegetables such as alaria, arame, bladderwrack, chlorella, nori, dulse, ecklonia cava, Irish moss, kelp, kombu, spirulina & wakame (can eat, powder form or supplement products).
- Coral calcium supplements.
- GABA - gamma aminobutyric acid is an amino acid that helps our body to relax, improve mental clarity, memory, moods, sleep and handle stress.
- Copper infused water - store water for 8 hours to overnight in 100% copper vessel, for instance a pitcher, mug or water bottle, and drink 1 to 2 glasses a day for its anti-inflammatory, antibacterial and antiviral properties.
- Detox vegetable tea - produce suggestions include burdock leaf, cabbage leaf, cilantro leaf, collard green, dandelion green, fennel leaf, garlic clove, ginger root, horseradish root, kale, leek, mustard green, onion, parsley leaf & turnip green. Simmer in gallon of water as many ingredients that you have available for about 30 minutes. Strain and drink cup of warm or cold tea 2 to 4 times a day. Keep in refrigerator for up to 1 week.
- Tamarind tea detox - bring 6 cups of water with 5 to 10 cut in half tamarind pods to a boil and simmer for 30 minutes. Remove pods and

drink ½ cup of hot, room temperature or cold tea 2 to 4 times a day. Keep in refrigerator for up to 1 week.
- Watermelon Cleanse, *Essiac Tea* or *Master Cleanse* (see Colon/Cleanses).
- Bentonite clay water (see Bentonite Clay).
- Possible B6, B12 and/or folate deficiency (see Minerals & Vitamins).
- Helps many people to balance hormones (see Hormone Imbalance).

Herbal Help
- Powdered greens (see Powdered Greens).
- Drink green tea 1 to 3 cups daily.
- Spirulina and/or chlorella products.
- Medical marijuana/cannabis products.

Herbs to Benefit the Brain
Amla berry, ashwagandha, bacopa, brahmi, fo-ti, ginkgo biloba, ginseng, gotu kola, holy basil, mung bean powder, periwinkle, rhodiola, rosemary, sage, turmeric and vacha

My Favorite Herbal Brain Combination
Ashwagandha, fo-ti, ginkgo biloba, gotu kola & turmeric

Take herbs in powdered, tincture, capsule or tea form - use any combination.

Some Causes & What Makes it Worse
- Dehydration & malnutrition.
- Hormonal imbalance.
- High sugar diet, such as a lot of white sugar, artificial sugar, high fructose corn syrup and all kinds of soda, sports drinks, energy drinks or alcohol.
- Limit or eliminate bad carbohydrates as much as possible, such as white flour products, pastas, breads, cakes, pies, donuts, french fries or chips.
- Chemical household and personal products, such as weed and bug poisons, cleaning supplies, detergents, toothpastes, deodorants or air fresheners.
- Food additives, such as preservatives, flavor enhancers, stabilizers or food coloring.
- Chronic stress can cause premature aging of the brain by releasing too much cortisol.
- Heavy metal accumulation or radiation exposure.
- Limit cell phone use or use protector to help reduce any harmful radiation.

- Cigarette smoking is known to thicken the blood and reduce oxygen supply to the brain which can make it harder to concentrate, focus and retain information.
- Some vaccinations are known to contain heavy metals, preservatives, formaldehydes, sugars, artificial colors or antibiotics.

BLOOD SUGAR IMBALANCE (PANCREAS)

The pancreas is a exocrine glandular organ located behind the stomach next to small intestine. The pancreas excretes enzymes to break down proteins and carbs. It secretes the hormone insulin to maintain healthier blood sugar levels.

In the year 1700 the average American consumed maybe 5 pounds of sugar a year; in the year 1900 about 90 pounds a year; and today it's up to 170 pounds a year. A 12 ounce can of soda equals about 9 to 12 packets or teaspoons of sugar.

General Symptoms of Imbalanced Blood Sugar Levels
- Line crease on earlobe.
- Weight gain or hard time losing weight.
- Blurry vision, flashes of light or eye floaters.
- Feeling sluggish in the morning.
- Fatigue, cranky, anxious or confused.
- Slow healing of cuts and wounds.
- Inner shakiness or twitching.
- Pain in pancreas area.
- Hormone imbalance, erectile dysfunction or loss of sexual desire.
- Loss of hair on lower extremities.
- Frequent yeast, fungal and bacterial infections.
- Craving sweets and caffeine.
- High blood pressure or high cholesterol.
- Increased sweating or urinate often.
- Fruity smell to breath and sweat.
- Wake up often while sleeping, when blood sugar drops at night.
- Headaches, poor memory, seizures, depression and/or panic attacks.
- Hard dark pigment in armpit, neck and/or groin.
- Jaundice or pale, pasty, yellowish complexion is when color of skin and whites of eyes turn yellow or pale orange.

- High blood sugar levels cause the body to lose fluids faster resulting in unusual, excessive thirst and dry skin, eyes or mouth.
- High blood sugar levels can make the blood pH acidic, which will pull calcium and minerals out of the bones to help balance pH. This could lead to bone mineral deficiency or weakened cartilage and tendons.
- Circulation issues such as muscle inflammation can cut off circulation in arms, legs and feet. Some nerves travel through the inflamed muscles. This can manifest as shooting pain, tingling, coldness, numbness and swelling.
- Women who wear a D cup bra or larger by age 20 are one and half times more likely to develop type 2 diabetes.
- Diabetes, cataracts, glaucoma, neuropathy and foot ulcers.

Natural Suggestions to Help Balance Blood Sugar Levels
- Physical activity - 3 times a week or more. Suggestions are walking, biking, gardening, stretching, light hand weights, swimming, dancing, yoga, tai chi or qigong. Physical activity stimulates the liver to release stored glucose sending signals to the brain to stop cravings for sugar and to help blood circulate throughout the body.
- Relax - suggestions are slow down, manage your stress level, listen to calming music, get plenty of sleep, do meditation, walk labyrinths and find some alone time.
- Switch to natural household and personal care products or make your own DIY products.
- Stones & crystals - amethyst, carnelian, citrine, sodalite or tiger's eye. Carry with you or on you, as jewelry, in your pocket, in your purse or lie down with stones on middle of back.
- Essential oils & reflexology to benefit the pancreas - anise, black pepper, dill, cinnamon, coriander fennel, geranium, ginger, grapefruit, helichrysum, juniper, lemon, ocotea, peppermint or rose. Choose your own blend and use in a spray, roll-on, eye pillow, diffuser, car diffuser, bath salts, body oil, massage oil or lotion. Mix 3 to 10 drops of essential oils in 1 to 3 tablespoons any carrier oil & massage the middle of back where pancreas is located and the arch of both feet, or massage arch of feet using foot roller or ball.

Internally
- Eat healthier (avoid or limit all sugars) & drink plenty of water. Good to eat protein in the mornings.
- Whole food blender drink daily - ingredient suggestions are almond, beet, bitter melon, broccoli, cabbage, carrot, celery, chaga mushroom, cherry,

chia seeds, curry leaf, green stevia leaf, kale, reishi mushroom, spinach, sprouts and swiss chard.

- About 30% of our daily food intake should be fiber foods. Fiber suggestions include apple pectin, barley, beans, chia seeds, farro, flaxseed meal, hemp hearts, konjac root, lentils, nuts, seeds, oats, peas, psyllium husks, sprouted breads, quinoa, fruits and vegetables.
- Eggs - best to look for pasture raised, cage free or free range.
- Use a good mineral filled sea salt instead of white table salt.
- Try a sweetener that is safer for diabetics such stevia, flavored stevia extract or xylitol powder.
- Possible chromium deficiency (see Minerals & Vitamins).
- Drink lemon water first thing in morning on an empty stomach.
- Garlic - swallow 1 to 3 chopped cloves like a pill or as a tincture, tea or pill supplement.
- Apple cider vinegar - 1 to 2 tablespoons in glass of water or herbal tea 1 to 3 times a day or before a high carbohydrate meal.
- White mulberry tea, pill supplement or dried fruit.
- Omega fatty acids.
- Cod liver oil or pill supplement.
- Mushroom supplement products or tea.
- Kombucha mushroom tea; buy or make.
- Bitter melon supplement products.
- Sea vegetables such as alaria, arame, bladderwrack, chlorella, nori, dulse, ecklonia cava, Irish moss, kelp, kombu, spirulina & wakame (can eat, powder form or supplement products).
- Coral calcium supplements.
- Healthy complex carbs including bran cereal, buckwheat, chia seeds, fruits, oatmeal, muesli, nuts, quinoa, seeds and vegetables.
- Alpha lipoic acid rich food sources are beet, brewer's yeast, broccoli, brussel sprout, carrot, collard green, organ meats, peas, red meats, spinach, Swiss chard, tomato and yam. Alpha lipoic acid is a fatty acid to convert glucose into energy.
- Anthocyanin rich foods sources (red-blue pigment produce) are acai berry, aronia berry, avocado, beet, bilberry, blackberry, blackcurrant, blueberry, blue tomato, cherry, cranberry, eggplant, elderberry, fig, grape, mango, olives, onion, plum, pomegranate seed, prune, purple sweet potato, radish, raspberry, strawberry and red cabbage Anthocyanins have antioxidant and anti-inflammatory properties.
- Raw pancreas glandular pill supplement.
- Watermelon Cleanse, *Essiac Tea* or *Master Cleanse* (see Colon/Cleanses).

Herbal Help
- Powdered greens (see Powdered Greens).
- Ground fenugreek seed tea - 1 teaspoon ground fenugreek seeds with a dropper of a flavored stevia extract.
- Cinnamon powder tea - 1 teaspoon cinnamon, 1 tablespoon raw honey and juice of half lemon.
- Take 1 capsule of cayenne or cinnamon with each meal or ¼ teaspoon added to glass of water.
- Yellow dock root decoction (see Herbs/Tea).
- Green tea with green stevia leaves and ½ teaspoon cinnamon powder.

Herbs to Help Balance Blood Sugar Levels
Astragalus, banaba, bilberry, bitter melon, cayenne, Chinese goldthread, cinnamon, curry leaf, duhat, fenugreek, garcinia cambogia, ginger, goat's rue, goldenseal, green stevia, gymnema sylvestre, hibiscus, holy basil, horsetail, jambul fruit or seed, licorice root, marshmallow root, milk thistle, panax ginseng, sage, schizandra, shilajit, skullcap, sumac, tamarind, turmeric, velvet bean and white mulberry

- Bitter melon reduces levels of glucose from the blood to lower blood sugar levels and promotes insulin production. Also helps to lower blood pressure and body temperature.
- Cinnamon helps balance blood sugar levels and slows the emptying of the stomach to reduce blood sugar spikes after a meal.
- Fenugreek nudges the pancreas to make digestive enzymes and appetite suppressant.
- Green stevia promotes insulin production to lower blood sugar levels, lower blood pressure, helps curb cravings and improves bone density.
- Gymnema sylvestre helps curb cravings, helps balance blood sugar levels, stimulates the growth of beta cells in the pancreas, rebuilds the pancreas and reduces hyperactivity.

My Favorite Herbal Blood Sugar Combination
Bitter melon, cinnamon, fenugreek, green stevia, gymnema sylvestre & turmeric

Take herbs in powder, tincture, capsule or tea form - use any combination.

Dried Herbal Blood Sugar Tea Combination
- Crushed Cinnamon Stick
- Curry Leaf
- Fenugreek Leaf
- Gymnema Sylvestre
- Hibiscus Leaf
- Holy Basil Leaf

- Green Stevia Leaf
- Turmeric Root

Use all above ingredients or any above dried herbal combination.

Mix ingredients together and store in closed container. 1 tablespoon dried herbal combination in small press n' brew empty tea bags, tea ball or mesh strainer per cup of hot water. Steep for 15 to 30 minutes and drink 1 to 3 cups a day.

Some Causes & What Makes it Worse
- High sugar diet, such as a lot of white sugar, artificial sugar, high fructose corn syrup and all kinds of soda, sports drinks, energy drinks or alcohol. Sugars suppress the immune system and contributes to the inflammation of muscles, tendons, cartilage and nerves.
- Limit or eliminate bad carbohydrates as much as possible, such as white flour products, pastas, breads, cakes, pies, donuts, cookies, french fries or chips. Refined white flour and breads are heavily refined and processed wheat grains stripped of their fiber and wheat germ nutrition leaving only simple carbohydrates. Basically, it becomes a form of sugar and has added chemicals to make it whiter and to last longer on shelves. The average American will eat 140 pounds of flour a year, but note two slices of white bread can equal 10 teaspoons of sugar.
- Food additives, such as preservatives, flavor enhancers, stabilizers or food coloring.
- Chemical household and personal products, such as weed and bug poisons, cleaning supplies, detergents, toothpastes, deodorants or air fresheners.
- Hydrogenated oils or trans fatty acids such as meat drippings, chicken skin, margarine, lard, microwave popcorn or store bought frosting.
- Cigarette smoking will increase blood sugar levels by as much as 30% followed by a quick drop after the cigarette is put out which could explain why you might crave that next cigarette.
- Long term infection, candida, fungal or bacterial infection.
- Lack of physical movement and being overweight.
- Some medications, such as birth control pills, diuretics, statins or steroids.

COLON HEALTH

The colon, also called the large intestine, is the last part of the digestive system. The small intestine's job is absorbing about 90% of nutrients and minerals from our food. While the colon or large intestine's job is to absorb small remaining amounts of nutrients, regulate flora and reabsorb fluids from digested food to form stools for elimination through the anus. It's important to clear the colon of old toxic stagnant stool. We should be eliminating (#2) about three times a day, but at least once a day.

Natural Suggestions for More Efficient Colon
- Physical activity - 3 times a week or more. Suggestions are walking, biking, gardening, swimming, dancing, stretching, yoga, tai chi or qigong.
- If you have to go, then GO. The longer stools stay in colon, the more the fluid is reabsorbed in the colon making the stools harder.
- Relax into yoga "child's resting pose" hold for about 2 to 5 minutes daily. Deep breathing while in pose helps massage internal organs.
- Slow down while eating; should chew about 20 times per bite. Taking big bites and eating fast increases the amount of air you swallow which can make you gassy and bloated.
- Colon hydrotherapy or colonics.
- Switch to natural household and personal care products or make your own DIY products.
- Avoid antibiotics, artificial sugars, chemical additives, chocolate, excessive caffcinc, large amounts of dairy, processed foods, all pain killers, over use of harsh laxatives, sugars, sugary drinks and foods.
- Squatting position stool, instead of standard sitting helps eliminate feces more easily, such as a *Squat Stool* or *Squatty Potty.*

Internally
- Eat healthier & drink a whole food blender drink daily - consider including some of the foods listed below.
- Drink plenty of water - at least half your body weight in ounces daily to hydrate the colon to prevent dry bulky hard stools. Good to drink 16 ounces of warm water first thing in the morning, drinking warm herbal teas throughout the day also help.
- About 30% of our daily food intake should be fiber foods. Fiber helps to move stool through the digestive tract and colon. Fiber suggestions include apple pectin, barley, beans, chia seeds, farro, flaxseed meal, hemp

hearts, konjac root, lentils, nuts, seeds, oats, peas, psyllium husks, sprouted breads, quinoa, fruits and vegetables.
- Leave on skins when possible, which is where a lot of the fiber is located.
- Plant based digestive enzyme pill supplements like papain from papaya and bromelain from pineapple.
- Enzyme rich food & drink sources include apple cider vinegar, apricot, avocado, bee pollen, coconut water, fermented vegetables, grape, kefir, kimchi, kiwi, kombucha mushroom tea, kvass, mango, melons, natto powder, papaya, pineapple, raw dairy products, raw honey, sauerkraut, water kefir, wheatgrass juice and yogurt.
- Digestive enzyme pill supplements including lipase, protease and amylase.
- Possible magnesium & potassium deficiency (see Minerals & Vitamins).
- Probiotics such as probiotic supplements such as acidophilus, or *Good Belly* drink or *Innergy Biotic* drink.

Natural Suggestions to Help with Constipation
- Enemas - an injection of liquid through the anus to promote elimination of the colon.
- Essential oils & reflexology to improve colon health - basil, black pepper, fennel, ginger, lavender, lemon, marjoram, orange, peppermint, pine, rosemary, spearmint or spruce. Mix 3 to 10 drops of essential oils of choice in 1 to 3 tablespoons any carrier oil & massage abdomen clockwise, feet or massage arch of both feet using foot roller or ball.

Internally
- Aloe vera gel scraped from leaf - 1 tablespoon 3 times a day after meals
- Apple cider vinegar drink - 1 tablespoon each of apple cider vinegar and raw honey in glass of warm water; stir and drink 1 to 3 times a day.
- *Natural Calm* is a powdered magnesium supplement known to help relax muscles, promote sleep and helps prevent muscle twitching, leg cramps and constipation.

Drink first thing in the morning on an empty stomach:
- 16 to 20 ounces of water or lemon water; colon could be just dry and unable to move through.
- Glass of prune juice.
- ¼ cup of sole water, castor oil or extra virgin olive oil.
- 1 to 3 tablespoons of baking soda or Epsom salts (magnesium sulfate) in a glass of water and follow with a quart of water within a couple of hours
- Bentonite clay water (see Bentonite Clay).

- 1 tablespoon whole flaxseeds in glass of water; let sit overnight and drink.

Eat:
- ½ dozen dried figs; soaked overnight in water. In the morning, drink the water and eat the figs.
- Banana, orange or a few prunes after each meal.
- 1 cup plain air popped popcorn.
- ½ cup strawberries, blueberries and/or raspberries or dried fruit.

Herbal Help
- Powdered greens (see Powdered Greens).
- Mix 1 teaspoon slippery elm bark powder in glass of water or juice.
- *Smooth Move Tea* or senna leaf tea.
- Yellow dock root decoction (see Herbs/Tea)
- *Springreen #77 Bentonite Detoxificant & #79 Intestinal Cleaner*

Herbs that Help with Constipation & Cleanse the Colon
Acai berries, aloe vera, apple pectin, cascara sagrada, cayenne, chaparral, fennel, flaxseeds, ginger, grapefruit pectin, licorice root, lobelia, malva leaf, marshmallow root, oregano, papaya leaf, pau d'arco, peppermint, psyllium husk, rhubarb root, senna, shatavari, slippery elm bark, tamarind, triphala and wormwood

- Cascara sagrada acts as a laxative and helps strengthen walls of the colon.
- Senna acts as a laxative to stimulate peristaltic movement of the digestive tract for better elimination.
- Slippery elm bark soothes the lining of the intestine and helps with diarrhea and constipation.
- Psyllium husks helps bulk up stool and activate bowel movements.

Take herbs in powdered, tincture, capsule or tea form - use any combination.

Herbal Powder Fiber Combination
Fennel seed powder, flaxseed powder, psyllium husk powder & slippery elm bark powder - use equal amounts of each

Mix powders together and store in closed container. 1 teaspoon to 1 tablespoon of powder in glass of water or juice; stir and drink; or encapsulate and take 2 to 4 capsules with 10 to 20 ounces of water.

Herbal Powder Laxative Combination

Aloe vera powder, cascara sagrada powder, chaparral powder, senna powder & slippery elm bark powder - use equal amounts of each

Mix powders together and store in closed container. 1 teaspoon to 1 tablespoon powder in glass of water or juice; stir and drink; or encapsulate and take 2 to 4 capsules with 10 to 20 ounces of water.

Dried Herbal Colon Cleanse Tea Combination
- Cascara Sagrada Bark
- Chamomile Flower
- Chaparral Leaf
- Flaxseed Meal
- Papaya Leaf
- Peppermint Leaf
- Psyllium Husk
- Senna Leaf

Use all above ingredients or any above dried herbal combination.

Mix ingredients together and store in closed container. 1 tablespoon of combination in small press n' brew empty tea bags, tea ball or mesh strainer per cup of hot water. Steep for 15 to 30 minutes and drink 1 to 3 cups at night before bed.

CLEANSES

Essiac Tea - (was discovered by Rene Caisse, a Canadian nurse. Essiac is Caisse spelled backwards) is called a tea but is actually a decoction which is a strong hot herbal tea. Uses four herbs, which you can buy the tea already made or buy the herbs already mixed. Make & take as directed on label.

Herbs in *Essiac Tea*:
- Burdock root is a blood and liver purifier, known to dissolve kidney stones, shrink tumors and help prevent them from growing.
- Rhubarb root is anti-inflammatory, antibacterial and is beneficial for digestive issues.
- Sheep sorrel is a natural antioxidant and good for stomach pains, known to shrink tumors and protects cells from damage.
- Slippery elm bark is a natural antioxidant and has a high mucilage content to help cleanse colon. Also beneficial for diarrhea and constipation.

Master Cleanse - (a liquid diet cleanse developed by Stanley Burroughs)
Combine all ingredients in a glass and make more as needed throughout day.
This is what you would drink all day and no other food or drink, except water or
herbal teas for up to 10 days. About 6 to 12 glasses daily. Do the best you can; I
was thrilled to do 3 days.

Ingredients:
- 8 to 10 ounces of spring or purified water
- Juice of ½ to whole lemon
- 2 tablespoons of maple syrup
- Pinch or two of cayenne pepper powder to taste

Some benefits of *Essiac Tea* and *Master Cleanse*:
- Known to help cleanse and strengthen the colon, liver, kidneys, heart, pancreas, bladder, glands, digestive system and lymph nodes to better perform their duties.
- Helps eliminate waste and hardened material in joints and muscles.
- Is known to reduce inflammation and pain .
- Strengthen immune system.
- Helps remove heavy metals, candida and parasites.
- Known to help maintain cholesterol and blood sugar levels.

Watermelon Cleanse - best to do in the summer when watermelons are in
season. Drinking watermelon juice is a good whole body cleanse which acts as a
natural diuretic to flush out toxins and trapped fluid, which improves
inflammation and circulation. And also helps cleanse organs such as the colon,
kidneys, liver, heart and bladder.
- Small whole watermelon.
- Blend and grind up the whole thing including the rind.
- Drink at night over a few hours before going to bed.
- If blender is not strong enough to blend rind, blend all but the outer rind.

HAPPY HEART

The heart is an organ about the size of your fist composed of muscle to pump blood throughout the body bringing oxygen and nutrients to organs and tissues.

Blood pressure is determined by how much blood your heart pumps and how much resistance to the blood flow is in your arteries. The more blood that your heart pumps and the narrower your arteries, the higher your blood pressure. Ideal blood pressure numbers are 115/120 over 75/80.

Good cholesterol (HDL) is a fat-like substance responsible for removing bad cholesterol and helping to produce vitamin D. Assists the body in digesting fat and is needed to form myelin to insulate nerve cells. Too much bad cholesterol (LDL) slowly builds up on the inner walls of the arteries to form plaque that can restrict circulation within the arteries.

General Symptoms of High Blood Pressure
- Red and/or large tip of nose.
- Shortness of breath.
- Hard to touch toes when bend over.
- Jaw, neck, arm and shoulder pain.
- Ear noise or ringing in the ear.
- Nosebleeds and red flushing of skin.
- Weak hand grip.
- Internal body heat rises.
- Vertical lines on side of ear.
- Swollen ankles, feet and lower legs.
- Unclear thinking, forgetfulness and difficulty concentrating.
- Warm and painful palms.
- Mood swings, irrational behavior.
- Prominent temporal vein.
- Pitting edema is when an indent is left in the skin after pushing on skin with fingers or from wearing socks and shoes.
- Shiny skin or red feet when standing and pale feet when elevated.

General Symptoms of High Cholesterol
- Line crease on earlobe.
- Depression and feeling sluggish or lack of energy.
- Yawning a lot, jaw pain.
- Shortness of breath.
- High blood sugar levels.
- Tend to gain excess belly weight.

- Plaque causes inflammation, which can lead to arm and leg pain.
- Mosquitoes tend to be attracted to you.
- Develop moles usually on arms, neck, legs and belly.
- Pain or numbness in legs - arteries that supply blood to legs could have narrowed.
- Develop yellowish thick patches or lumps called xanthomas, especially around the eyes, eyelids and hands.

Signs of having heart attack - seek medical help for following symptoms:
- Shortness of breath.
- Cold sweat and unusual fatigue.
- Dizziness or light headed when blood pressure drops too low.
- Pain or tightness in the neck, jaw, chest and arms.
- Nausea, bad heartburn or stomach pain.

When having a heart attack - take cayenne or 2 aspirin as soon as possible. This has been known to help, at least until medical assistance arrives:
- 1 teaspoon of cayenne powder stirred in glass of warm water and drink.
- 3 to 6 squirts of cayenne alcohol tincture.
- Pinch of cayenne powder on tongue.

Natural Suggestions to Improve Heart Health
- Physical activity - 3 times a week or more. Suggestions are walking, biking, gardening, stretching, light hand weights, swimming, dancing, yoga, tai chi or qigong. When you exercise, you increase your circulation and the blood flow throughout your body.
- Relax to help lower blood pressure - suggestions are slow down, manage your stress level, get plenty of sleep, do meditation, walk labyrinths and find some alone time.
- Sound therapy to help lower blood pressure - listen to calming music, white noise, pink noise, electroencephalogram music, using tuning forks or singing bowls.
- Avoid tight fitting clothes, such as when socks leave an indent on legs when removed after a long period of time, when bra leaves an indent on back or pants leave indent on waist. These could affect blood pressure.
- Stand on your head for 2 to 10 minutes - inverted position is known to give the heart a break.
- Dry skin brushing increases circulation.
- Acupuncture, chiropractor or massage therapy.

- Stones & crystals - aventurine, jade, malachite, rose quartz or turquoise. Carry with you or on you, as jewelry, in your pocket, in your purse or lay down with stone on your heart. Place stone in bra under left breast.
- Essential oils & reflexology to benefit the heart - geranium, jasmine, juniper, lavender, neroli, nutmeg, rose, rosemary or ylang ylang. Choose your own blend and use in a spray, roll-on, eye pillow, diffuser, car diffuser, bath salts, body oil, massage oil or lotion. Mix 3 to 10 drops in 1 to 3 tablespoons any carrier oil & lightly massage between breasts and under both breasts. Also, massage arch of feet or massage arch of feet using foot roller or ball.

Internally
- Eat healthier & drink plenty of water.
- Powdered greens (see Powdered Greens).
- Whole food blender drink daily - ingredient suggestions are acai berry, apricot kernel, blueberry, chia seeds, flaxseed meal, ginger, goji berry, hemp heart, kale, lecithin, nuts, prune and spinach.
- Use a good mineral filled sea salt instead of white table salt.
- Garlic tincture - 1 squirt 2 to 3 times a day.
- Garlic - swallow 1 to 3 chopped garlic cloves like a pill, or as a tea or pill supplement.
- Eat 3 to 5 organic radishes a day (black, daikon, purple or red).
- Copper infused water - store water for 8 hours to overnight in 100% copper vessel, for instance a pitcher, mug or water bottle and drink 1 to 2 glasses a day for its anti-inflammatory, antibacterial and antiviral properties.
- Super fruit juices including acai, goji, mangosteen, noni or pomegranate.
- Cranberry concentrate - take 1 tablespoon 3 times a day.
- White mulberry tea, pill supplements or dried fruit.
- Grape seed extract supplement products.
- Non-GMO soy or lecithin products.
- CBD products.
- Natto powder.
- Possible potassium & magnesium deficiency (see Minerals & Vitamins).
- Food grade diatomaceous earth helps lower cholesterol. Stir 1 teaspoon to 1 tablespoon in water, juice, coconut water, aloe vera juice and drink daily.
- Red yeast rice is a natural statin, promotes blood circulation and can lower cholesterol levels.
- Coenzyme Q10 helps prevent blood clot formation.

- Sea vegetables such as alaria, arame, bladderwrack, chlorella, nori, dulse, ecklonia cava, Irish moss, kelp, kombu, spirulina & wakame (can eat, powder form or supplement products).
- Coral calcium supplements.
- Evening primrose oil - main ingredient is GLA (gamma linolenic acid), an essential fatty acid known to help prevent hardening of the arteries.
- Omega fatty acids.
- Quercetin is a flavonoid found in foods like buckwheat tea, green tea, apple, berries, kale, onion, red wine, pomegranate and St. John's Wort.
- Super Tonic (see DIY Recipes).
- Blood thinning foods like almond, apple, apricot, blueberry, cayenne pepper, cherry, cinnamon, dandelion green, garlic, ginger, grape, kale, grapefruit, peppers, olive oil, onion, orange, mint leaf, pineapple, prune, raisin, raw potato, spinach, strawberry, tangerine, tomato and turmeric.
- Healthy oils including avocado oil, extra virgin olive oil, grapeseed oil, sunflower oil and safflower oil.
- About 30% of our daily food intake should be fiber foods. Fiber suggestions include apple pectin, barley, beans, chia seeds, farro, flaxseed meal, hemp hearts, konjac root, lentils, nuts, seeds, oats, peas, psyllium husks, sprouted breads, quinoa, fruits and vegetables.
- Strive to balance blood sugar levels (see Blood Sugar Imbalance) - helps blood not to clot and lowering triglycerides levels.

My first choices to help lower blood pressure - drink 2 to 3 times a day:
- Apple cider vinegar drink - 1 tablespoon each of apple cider vinegar and raw honey in glass of warm water.
- Take a capsule each of cayenne & garlic pill supplements.
- Glass of lemon water with 1 teaspoon of powdered herb combination of cayenne, garlic, cinnamon, turmeric and ginger powder; stir and drink 1 to 3 times a day.
- Hibiscus & green tea.
- Cup of hot water with 1 tablespoon of cinnamon powder, 1 tablespoon of raw honey and dash of cayenne; stir and drink 2 to 3 times a day.

Herbs to Lower Blood Pressure
Astragalus, cayenne, cilantro, cinnamon, clove, cramp bark, ecklonia cava, garlic, ginger, ginkgo biloba, gotu kola, guggul, green tea, hawthorn berry, hibiscus, jasmine, jiaogulan, linden flowers, motherwort, nutmeg, olive leaf, rauwolfia, red clover, rehmannia, saffron, snakeroot, tamarind, tilia, wood betony and turmeric

Blood Thinning Herbs (USE WITH CAUTION IF TAKING BLOOD THINNING MEDICATION)
Cayenne, Chinese goldthread, danshen, devil's claw, dong quai, feverfew, garlic, ginkgo biloba, ginger, hibiscus, horse chestnut, pau d'arco, rosemary, skullcap, tamarind, turmeric and white willow bark

Herbs to Lower Cholesterol Levels
Alcachofa, alfalfa, apple pectin, banaba leaf, butcher's broom, cayenne, cinnamon, dill, ecklonia cava, fenugreek, garlic, ginger, guggul, hawthorn berry, hibiscus, holy basil, jasmine, jiaogulan, licorice root, milk thistle, olive leaf, oregano, red clover, sumac, thyme, turmeric and white mulberry

My Favorite Herbal Heart Health Combination
Cayenne, garlic, ginger, guggul, hawthorn berry & turmeric

Herbal High Blood Pressure Combination
Gotu kola, linden flower or tilia, hawthorn berry & rauwolfia

Take herbs in powdered, tincture, capsule or tea form - use any combination.

Dried Herbal Happy Heart Tea Combination
- Alcachofa Leaf
- Coriander Seed
- Crushed Cinnamon Stick
- Ginger Root
- Hawthorn Leaf or Berry
- Hibiscus Flower
- Holy Basil Leaf
- Rooibos Leaf

Use all above ingredients or any above dried herbal combination.

Mix ingredients together and store in closed container. 1 tablespoon dried herbal combination in small press n' brew empty tea bags, tea ball or mesh strainer per cup of hot water. Steep for 15 to 30 minutes and drink 1 to 3 cups a day.

Some Causes & What Makes it Worse
- Dehydration & malnutrition.
- High sugar diet, such as a lot of white sugar, artificial sugar, high fructose corn syrup and all kinds of soda, sports drinks, energy drinks or alcohol.
- Limit or eliminate bad carbohydrates as much as possible, such as white flour products, pastas, breads, cakes, pies, cookies, french fries or chips.
- Limit or eliminate use of white table salt, whose white color is due to bleaching and high processing. Contains dextrose and anti-caking agents to eliminate clumps and has a strong salty taste from the additives added.

- Limit or avoid processed and refined foods.
- Excessive red meat or caffeine consumption.
- Hydrogenated oils or trans fatty acids such as meat drippings, chicken skin, margarine, lard, microwave popcorn or store bought frosting.
- Chemical household and personal products, such as weed and bug poisons, cleaning supplies, detergents, toothpastes, deodorants or air fresheners.
- Cigarette smoking is known to raise blood pressure and heart rate while hardening and narrowing the walls of the arteries. If you quit smoking, your good LDL could improve quickly by 10%.
- Lack of physical movement and being overweight.
- Heavy metal accumulation.

HORMONE &THYROID IMBALANCE

Hormones are glands of our endocrine and exocrine systems and play a vital role in everyone's health and well-being. Hormones are chemical messengers created by the body. They transfer information from one set of cells to another in order to coordinate the functions of different parts of the body.

The major glands of the endocrine system are the adrenal glands, hypothalamus gland, ovaries, pancreas, parathyroid gland, pineal gland, pituitary gland, testes, thymus gland and thyroid gland. The exocrine system are glands that produce, secrete and transfer their product (e.g., breast milk, digestive bile, sweat and tears) through ducts. The major glands of the exocrine system are ceruminous glands, lacrimal glands, liver, mammary glands, mucous glands, pancreas, salivary glands, sebaceous glands and sweat glands.

We probably all have had some symptoms of hormone imbalance which we have come to believe are "normal." When hormones fluctuate, it can affect your moods, instigate depression, headaches and irrational thinking. They influence bone growth, regulate metabolism and known to affect sleeping patterns. The imbalance of hormones may impact negatively on how your reproductive system works including low sexual desire, infertility, menopause symptoms and much more. Women of all ages experience hormonal imbalances. Children and men are also affected by imbalance of hormones.

General Symptoms for Unbalanced Hormones
- Impatient and anxiety.
- Mood swings, depression and talk very slow.
- Excessive crying, angry and low self esteem.

- Eating disorders, addictions and being very obsessive.
- Memory loss, brain fog, migraines and autism.
- Thin brittle nails or chew fingernails.
- Red chin, acne and dry skin.
- Problems sleeping, feeling tired or not waking feeling refreshed in morning.
- Need to take naps during day.
- Unexplained weight gain or weight loss.
- Inability to lose weight.
- Weakened bones, muscle weakness, joint pain and arthritis.
- Loss of muscle tone or bone loss.
- Poor social skills or hyperactive.
- Low sex drive or excessive sex drive.
- Thinning hair or excessive hair on body.
- Body is unusually small or large in size.

Additional symptoms for women:
- Heavy menstrual bleeding, PMS, bloating, painful periods, vaginal dryness and tender breasts.
- Hard time getting pregnant.
- Water retention, bloating and vaginal infections.
- Hot flashes and night sweats.
- Lactating when not pregnant.
- Thick, hard skin areas on ball of one or both feet can be connected to the breasts.

Additional symptoms for men:
- Prostate and testicular issues.
- Develop breast tissue.
- Low sperm count.
- Erectile dysfunction.

Natural Suggestions to Balance Hormones
- Physical activity - 3 times a week or more. Suggestions are walking, biking, gardening, stretching, swimming, dancing, yoga, tai chi or qigong.
- Get enough sleep at night, in bed by 10pm can prevent throwing hormones into overdrive.
- Relax - suggestions are slow down, manage your stress level, listen to calming music, massage therapy, do meditation, walk labyrinths and find some alone time.
- Occasional day of fasting to help clean system of toxins.
- Acupuncture, chiropractic or reflexology.

- Switch to natural household and personal care products or make your own DIY products.
- Wild yam cream or gel.
- Evening primrose oil cream.
- Hyperbaric oxygen therapy.
- Stones & crystals - amber, carnelian, citrine, jade, malachite, moonstone, lapis, sodalite or quartz. Carry with you or on you, as jewelry, in your pocket, in your purse or bra or jade eggs for toning vagina.
- Essential oils & reflexology to assist hormone function - bergamot, birch, cedarwood, chamomile, clary sage, frankincense, geranium, grapefruit, lavender, lemon balm, myrtle, neroli, nutmeg, orange, peppermint, rose, sage, sandalwood, spearmint, thyme or ylang ylang. Choose your own blend and use in a spray, roll-on, eye pillow, diffuser, car diffuser, bath salts, body oil, massage oil or lotion. Mix 3 to 10 drops in 1 to 3 tablespoons of evening primrose oil, borage oil or any carrier oil & massage breasts, under arms, neck and abdomen. Massage both feet, ankles, and top of feet 1 to 3 times a day.
- Make herbal hormonal oil, salve or cream using herbal combination. Herb suggestions include black cohosh, chaste tree berries, damiana, sage, red raspberry or wild yam. Uses include rubbing into abdomen, breasts, face, feet, ankles, inner thigh, neck, scalp, testicles, upper inner arms and vagina area or where needed (see Herbs/Oils/Salves).

Internally
- Eat healthier & drink plenty of water.
- Powdered greens (see Powdered Greens).
- Whole food blender drink daily - ingredient suggestions are almond, beet, black radish, blueberry, cabbage, cordycep, evening primrose oil, ghee, goji berry, kale, kiwi, maca root or powder, pomegranate seed, pumpkin seed, raw honey, red raspberry leaf, reishi mushroom, spinach and turmeric root.
- If you drink milk it's best to look for whole milk without artificial growth hormones and pasture raised, cage free or free range eggs.
- Flaxseeds or omega fatty acids - to help repair hormone receptor sites.
- Evening primrose oil, borage oil or blackcurrant oil - ingest oil or put oil into empty capsules or take pill supplement.
- Apple cider vinegar drink - 1 tablespoon each of apple cider vinegar and raw honey in glass of warm water; stir and drink 1 to 3 times a day.
- Pine pollen products - helps strengthen immune system, increases energy, stamina and libido. Boosts testosterone levels, improves fertility and breast health.

- Bone broth, gelatin or collagen powder - best to look for grass-fed, pasture raised or organic.
- Non-GMO soy or lecithin products.
- Medical marijuana/cannabis products.
- DHEA products - is a hormone produced by the adrenal glands and reaches maximum levels around the age 25 then decreases as we get older
- Sea vegetables such as alaria, arame, bladderwrack, chlorella, nori, dulse, ecklonia cava, Irish moss, kelp, kombu, spirulina & wakame (can eat, powder form or supplement products).
- Coral calcium supplements.
- Herbal hormone balancing sprays.
- Watermelon Cleanse, *Essiac Tea* or *Master Cleanse* (see Colon/Cleanses).
- Some good herbal supplement products online are *Gaia - Woman's Balance, Nature's Answer - Female Complex* or *Herbally Grounded - Balance, My Secret, Replenish, Restore and Might For Men.*

Dried Herbal Hormone Balance Tea Combination

- Blessed Thistle Leaf
- Chamomile Flower
- Chaste Tree Berry
- Damiana Leaf
- Nettle Leaf
- Red Raspberry Leaf
- Sage Leaf
- Saw Palmetto Berry

Use all above ingredients or any above dried herbal combination. Mix ingredients together and store in closed container. Put 1 teaspoon to 1 tablespoon dried herbal combination in small press n' brew empty tea bags, tea ball or mesh strainer per cup of boiling water. Steep for 15 to 30 minutes and drink 1 to 3 cups a day.

Herbs to Balance Hormones for Women

Alfalfa grass, ashwagandha, black cohosh, blessed thistle, blue cohosh, catuaba bark, chaste tree berries or vitex, cramp bark, damiana, dong quai, false unicorn, fenugreek, hibiscus, horny goat weed or barrenwort, kudzu, maca, motherwort, mung bean, nettle, oat grass, panax ginseng, rehmannia, red clover, red raspberry, sage, sarsaparilla, saw palmetto, schizandra, shatavari, suma root, squaw vine, tongkat ali, turmeric, velvet bean, wild yam and yohimbe.

- Black cohosh helps prevent menstrual cramps, hot flashes, mood swings, menopause symptoms, vaginal dryness and helps stimulate labor.
- Blessed thistle helps with PMS, increases breast milk production and improve digestion.

- Chaste tree berries or vitex is a general hormone balancing herb, mood swings, hot flashes, vaginal dryness and endometriosis, fertility enhancer, cramps, bloating, breast tenderness and increases breast milk production.
- Damiana is a general hormone balancing, fertility enhancer and increases libido.
- Dong quai helps with PMS, menstrual cramps, irregular menstruation and hot flashes.
- Maca root is a general hormone balancing herb, increases libibdo, fertility enhancer, mood swings, PMS and hot flashes.
- Red raspberry is a gentle but powerful herb to gently balance hormones, my favorite herb for kids or when pregnant. Known to improve irregular menstruation, fertility enhancer, mood swings, cramps and brain function. Like alfalfa & nettle, red raspberry has a high mineral and vitamin content.
- Sage is helpful to prevent painful periods, hot flashes and excessive sweating, improves brain function, grey hair and hair restoration.
- Saw palmetto is a general hormone balancing herb, fertility enhancer, mood swings, vaginal dryness, irregular menstruation, heavy bleeding, breast enhancement, hair restoration, improves menopause symptoms and brain function and increases libido.
- Turmeric helps supports postmenopausal symptoms, menstrual cramps and increases circulation.
- Wild yam is a general hormone balancing herb, hot flashes, fertility enhancer and menstrual cramps.
- Yohimbe causes natural release of adrenalin to help with anxiety, benefits erectile dysfunction, increases blood flow, libido and stamina.

My Favorite General Hormone Balancing Combination - chaste tree berry, damiana, dong quai, maca, nettle, saw palmetto & wild yam

My Favorite Stop Hot Flashes/Menopause Combination - black cohosh, blue cohosh, dong quai, maca, red clover & sage.

My Favorite Combination to Increase Breast Milk Production - blessed thistle, fenugreek, goat's rue, motherwort & red raspberry.

Take herbs in powdered, tincture, capsule or tea form - use any combination.

Herbs to Balance Hormones for Men
Ashwagandha, catuaba bark, coleus forskohlii, chuan xiong, damiana, dong quai, eleuthero root, fenugreek, fu pen zi, horny goat weed, jiaogulan, lu rong (deer

antler), lu jiao shuang (deer antler), maca, muira puama, nettle, pine bark, red clover, red raspberry, rehmannia, sarsaparilla, saw palmetto, shatavari, Siberian ginseng, suma root, tongkat ali, tribulus terrestris, velvet bean and yohimbe.

My Favorite Herbal General Hormone Balancing Combination for Men
Ashwagandha, damiana, maca, nettle, saw palmetto & tribulus terrestris.

My Favorite Herbal Combination to Increase Libido
Fenugreek, horny goat weed, Lu rong & yohimbe.

My Favorite Herbal Prostate Health Combination for Men
Maca, nettle, pygeum & saw palmetto.

My Favorite Pregnancy & Children Herbal Combination
Alfalfa grass, blessed thistle, maca, motherwort, nettle & red raspberry. Take herbs in powdered, tincture, capsule or tea form.

Take herbs in powdered, tincture, capsule or tea form - use any combination.

Some Causes of Imbalanced Hormones & What Makes it Worse
- Bad eating habits will reduce production of testosterone, which helps with muscle strength, energy, mood regulation and sex drive.
- High sugar diet, such as a lot of white sugar, artificial sugar, high fructose corn syrup and all kinds of soda, sports drinks, energy drinks or alcohol.
- Limit or eliminate bad carbohydrates as much as possible, such as white flour products, pastas, breads, cakes, pies, donuts, french fries or chips.
- Hydrogenated oils or trans fatty acids such as meat drippings, chicken skin, margarine, lard, microwave popcorn or store bought frosting.
- Chemical household and personal products, such as weed and bug poisons, cleaning supplies, detergents, toothpastes, deodorants or air fresheners.
- Organophosphate is a pesticide used on fruits and vegetables and is known to lower testosterone levels.
- Triclosan found in some toothpaste and antibacterial soaps have been related to damaging sperm potency.
- Yeast and fungal overgrowth that can affect how the endocrine glands function.
- Plastics mimic estrogen in the body. Plastics numbered 3, 6 or 7 on bottom of products, should be eliminated as much as possible. Never microwave food in plastic or styrofoam. BPA is plastic used in lining of food cans, plastic containers and receipt paper.

- Parabens are chemicals used as synthetic preservatives to prevent mold and yeast. They are used as preservative in foods, pharmaceuticals and many commercial cosmetics, deodorants, toothpastes, hair and skin products. Can cause hormonal imbalance, skin issues or allergic reactions.
- Avoid non-stick coating or aluminum pots and pans; best to use stainless steel, cast iron, glass or ceramic.
- Cigarette smoking releases enzymes that lower testosterone levels.
- Antibiotics and artificial growth hormones are given to livestock to help make them grow bigger, fatter, produce more milk or eggs. Eating meat and dairy products containing artificial growth hormones is known to contribute to hormone imbalance, early puberty in girls, boys growing breast tissue, reproduction problems and breast, colon and prostate cancer. Best to eat organic or antibiotic and hormone free meats, poultry, fish, eggs and dairy products.
- Birth control pills, bioidenticals or any HRT (hormone replacement therapy) can lower testosterone levels, which makes the estrogen level too high. Birth control pills are known to cause weight gain, breast tenderness, nausea, headaches, mood changes and decreased libido. If you feel you have to take them, at least take herbs along with them for balance.
- Some medications such as acne medication, painkillers, heart medications, statins, anti-depression and hair loss medication or overuse of diet pills.
- Fluoride and chlorine are known to reduce production of iodine in body.
- Radiation, x-rays, heavy metal accumulation, pollution or smog.
- Bug sprays containing chlorpyrifos and sunscreens containing oxybenzone are both known to lower testosterone levels.
- Men should avoid tight fitting underwear as they can reduce sperm count and testosterone production. Better to wear loose fitting boxers.

THYROID IMBALANCE

The thyroid gland is butterfly shaped located on the front of the neck under the Adam's apple. The thyroid is known to help the body regulate body fat, body temperature, energy levels and much more.

General Symptoms of Thyroid Imbalance
- Enlargement of the neck or tongue.
- Two necklace lines or horizontal lines on neck where gland is located.

- Loss or thinning of outside of eyebrows.
- Dry rough skin, brittle nails, hair loss or thinning.
- Brain fog, forgetfulness and depression.
- Sensitivity to cold, especially hands and feet or having the chills.
- Chronic dehydration.
- Unexplained weight gain or weight loss.
- Always feeling tired and fatigued.
- Bulging eyes, double chin and puffy eyes, raspy voice.
- Chronic constipation, chronic diarrhea or irritable bowel syndrome.
- Excessive sweating and feeling overly warm.
- Hyperactive, jittery and feeling wired.
- Palms turned to the rear while standing with arms down at sides.
- Excess mucus, chronic sinus and throat issues.
- Chlorine and fluoride are known to block iodine receptors in the thyroid.
- Goiter, Graves' disease or Hashimoto.

Natural Suggestions for Thyroid Health

Many of us can balance the thyroid by balancing our hormones by using the suggestions listed above (see Natural Suggestions to Balance Hormones) since the thyroid is part of the endocrine system. However, some of us need to do more.

Here are some ideas:
- Lightly massage neck and lightly press hollow at base of the throat to stimulate thyroid. Press area 3 times for 5 seconds
- Rotate hot and cold packs on neck.
- Infrared LED light therapy - helps increase blood flow to injured tissues to help with acne, stretch marks, wrinkles, cellulite, excess pigment, scar tissue, sore muscles and organs.
- Essential oils & reflexology to assist thyroid function - anise, basil, cedarwood, clove, frankincense, geranium, grapefruit, lemon balm, myrrh, lemongrass, peppermint, rosemary or spearmint. Choose your own blend and use in a spray, roll-on, eye pillow, diffuser, bath salts or body oil. Mix 3 to 10 drops in 1 to 3 tablespoons evening primrose oil or any carrier oil & gently massage neck, feet, ankles and big toes 1 to 3 times a day.

Internally
- Possible iodine, copper or selenium deficiency (see Minerals & Vitamins).
- Sea vegetables are an excellent source of iodine, such as alaria, arame, bladderwrack, chlorella, dulse, ecklonia cava, Irish moss, kelp, kombu,

nori, spirulina & wakame (can eat, powder form or supplement products).
- Liquid iodine supplement.
- CBD products.
- Raw thyroid glandular pill supplement.

Herbs to Balance Thyroid
Ashwagandha, bacopa, black cohosh, black walnut hulls, bugleweed, coleus forskohlii, dandelion, echinacea, fennel, ginger, guggul, hyssop, lemon balm, maca, motherwort, nettle, prunella, red raspberry and rhodiola rosea

My Favorite Thyroid Combination
Bladderwrack, bugleweed, kelp & Irish moss

Take herbs in powdered, tincture, capsule form - use any combination.

INFLAMMATION, IMPROVED CIRCULATION & REDUCTION of PAIN

Inflammation and poor circulation can cause pain within the body. Many diseases are linked to inflammation including bursitis, colitis hepatitis, sinusitis, osteoporosis, tendonitis and tuberculosis. Inflammation is known to impact many health issues such as heart health, allergies, asthma, infections, diabetes, lupus and different kinds of arthritis.

General Symptoms of Inflammation & Poor Circulation
- Cold hands and feet.
- Chronic pain.
- Swelling, cramps, twitching or edema of hands, arms, feet and legs.
- Discoloration of skin like white, blue or slightly bruised.
- Varicose veins, fragile nails and hair loss.
- Erectile dysfunction can be caused by sluggish circulation.
- Hard to focus, poor memory and headaches.
- Your skin is dry even if drinking plenty of water.
- Shortness of breath and feeling tired.
- Loss of appetite and lowered immune system.
- Chest pain or heart attack.

Natural Suggestions to Help Relieve Inflammation
- Physical activity - 3 times a week or more. Suggestions are walking, biking, light hand weights, gardening, swimming, dancing, yoga, tai chi or qigong.
- Stretching daily increases circulation, blood flow to area, flexibility and range of motion.
- Massage therapies or massage tools (see Massage Therapy).
- Physical therapy.
- Foot reflexology or foot zoning.
- Acupuncture, chiropractic or reiki.
- EFT or Emotional Freedom Technique - a process of tapping areas of the body to clear out negative energy blockages. Helps with pain, stress, fear, inflammation, depression, anxiety and headaches. EFT is easy to learn and easy to do on yourself.
- Magnetic or copper therapy products.
- Wearing gold jewelry has been known to have healing properties.

- Infrared LED light therapy - helps increase blood flow to injured tissues to help with acne, stretch marks, wrinkles, cellulite, excess pigment, scar tissue, sore muscles and organs.
- Therapeutic ultrasound.
- Floatation tank therapy.
- Hyperbaric oxygen therapy.
- Biofeedback mat.
- Whole body cryotherapy.
- Inversion table has been known to help relieve back pain.
- Kinesiology tape - an elastic tape used for muscle, ligament and tendon pain relief.
- Foam roller, soft roller or body rolling.
- Menthol pain patches or capsaicin hot patches.
- Himalayan salt block or chunk - hold or lay sore area on salt block, put feet on top of blocks to help with pain and to detox body.
- TENS unit machine (transcutaneous electrical nerve stimulation unit).
- *Shao Lin* (electronic acupuncture apparatus).
- Sound therapy - *Vibroacoustic Therapy*, sound lounge bed and chairs.

Apply to sore area and leave on for 20 to 30 minutes and then off for 20 to 30 minutes, repeat as needed:
- Ice - the first thing I do for a bruised injury, painful area or inflammation is apply ice, for instance an ice bag, gel ice pack, bag of frozen peas or plastic storage bag filled with ice cubes. You can also use a paper cup filled with ice or wrap cloth around ice cube and rub cube into bruised or swollen area. The faster you get ice on the injury the better. Be careful not to fall asleep with ice on the area.
- Homemade gel ice pack - 1 cup of rubbing alcohol and 2 cups water in a gallon zip lock bag, double bag with as little air as possible. Place in freezer for about 2 hours before using.
- Frozen cabbage leaves.
- Rotate hot and cold therapy - to increase circulation; use heating pad or warm compress and rotate with ice pack, always end with cold.
- Warm compresses using castor oil, borage oil, mustard seed oil or warm sole water; soak a cotton, muslin or flannel cloth and apply (not on open wound). Can cover with plastic wrap or a towel and put heating pad or hot water bottle on top.
- Wet a brown paper bag or cloth with apple cider vinegar and then wrap around area.
- Warm baked potato pulp.

Rub gently onto sore areas 1 to 5 times a day:
- Menthol Salve (see DIY Recipes).
- Lobelia and/or St. John's wort oil (see Herbs/Oils).
- Garlic Oil (see DIY Recipes).
- Medical marijuana/cannabis products.
- CBD hemp oil products.
- Magnesium oil.
- Arnica products.
- Capsicum products.
- Mix raw honey & cinnamon powder into paste.
- Mix 1 tablespoon each of cayenne pepper powder & cinnamon powder with ½ cup extra virgin olive oil.
- Cayenne pepper oil - cut up 3 to 5 cayenne or red hot chili peppers, 2 cinnamon sticks and 2 inches of ginger root and mix with 2 cups of extra virgin olive oil. Simmer on stove for 20 to 30 minutes; allow to cool, strain and put oil into bottles.
- L-arginine cream or gel.
- DMSO products (dimethyl sulfoxide).
- Shark cartilage products.
- Buy or make pain herbal oil or salve using herbs such as cayenne, ginger, lobelia, medical marijuana and/or St. John's Wort. Optional to add arnica oil, menthol crystals and below essential oils (see Herbal/Oil/Salves).
- Essential oils & reflexology to improve inflammation & circulation - basil, birch, capsaicin, cedarwood, cinnamon, citronella, eucalyptus, frankincense, ginger, helichrysum, lavender, myrrh, oregano, peppermint, pine, spruce, rosemary or wintergreen. Mix 3 to 10 drops of essential oils of your choice in 1 to 3 tablespoons any carrier oil and massage into sore areas. Example pain combination - 2 drops each of capsaicin, eucalyptus, helichrysum & peppermint essential oils mixed with 2 tablespoons of extra virgin olive oil.
- Emu oil products.
- *Dit Da Jow* is an Asian liniment.
- Some homeopathic supplement products online are *Topricin* or *Triflora*.
- Some good menthol supplement products online are *Tiger Balm, CryoDerm, Soothanol S2, Polar Lotion, White Flower, Biofreeze* or *Zen Balm.*

Bath - add one of the following to your bath water; soak in warm to hot bath for about 15 to 45 minutes; suggestion to shower after to rinse off toxins:
- ½ cup to 1 cup bentonite clay, Epsom salt, ginger, magnesium powder, sea salt, sole water, apple cider vinegar or any combination.
- ½ cup to 2 cups Bath Powder Blend (see DIY Recipes).

- Foot baths - 2 tablespoons to ½ cup of any suggestion above.

Internally
- Eat healthier & drink plenty of water.
- Whole food blender drink daily - ingredient suggestions are almond, beet, blueberry, celery, cherry, chia seeds, collard green, garlic, ginger, kale, onion, papaya, peppers, pineapple, spinach, swiss chard, turmeric and walnut.
- Use a good mineral filled sea salt instead of white table salt.
- Garlic - swallow 1 to 3 chopped garlic cloves like a pill, or as a tincture, tea or pill supplement.
- Place golden raisins in a jar, cover raisins with gin and soak for 1 week; store soaked raisins in the refrigerator and eat 9 raisins a day. Helps with inflammation, pain and arthritis.
- Cherries help prevent crystallization of uric acid, reduce uric acid levels in the blood and helps knuckle bumps disappear. Eat a dozen a day, tart is better or drink sugar free cherry juice.
- Glass of lemon water with 1 teaspoon of powdered herb combination of cayenne, garlic, cinnamon, turmeric and ginger powder; stir and drink 1 to 3 times a day.
- Black cherry concentrate - take 1 tablespoon 3 times a day.
- Take 1 tablespoon of raw honey at each meal.
- Drink 1 cup of warm water and 1 tablespoon of blackstrap molasses daily.
- Apple cider vinegar - mix 1 tablespoon in a glass of water; 1 to 3 times a day. Helps remove calcium deposits to reduce inflammation against arthritis and bursitis.
- Apple cider vinegar drink - 1 tablespoon each of apple cider vinegar and raw honey in glass of warm water; stir and drink 1 to 3 times a day.
- Omega fatty acids help reduce inflammation.
- Drink bentonite clay water every day, and my personal favorite remedy for arthritis (see Bentonite Clay).
- Copper infused water - store water for 8 hours to overnight in 100% copper vessel, for instance a pitcher, mug or water bottle and drink 1 to 2 glasses a day for its anti-inflammatory, antibacterial and antiviral properties.
- Grape seed extract supplement products.
- Super Tonic (see DIY Recipes).
- Bone broth, gelatin or collagen powder - best to look for grass-fed, pasture raised or organic.

- Sea vegetables such as alaria, arame, bladderwrack, chlorella, nori, dulse, ecklonia cava, Irish moss, kelp, kombu, spirulina & wakame (can eat, powder form or supplement products).
- Coral calcium supplements.
- Quercetin is a flavonoid found in foods like buckwheat tea, green tea, apple, berries, kale, onion, pomegranate, red wine and St. John's Wort.
- Watermelon Cleanse (see Colon/Cleanses).
- MSM, magnesium or CBD hemp oil products.
- Glucosamine and chondroitin helps rebuild cartilage; especially good for arthritis and joint pain.

Herbal Help

- Cut up fresh ginger root and put in muslin bag. Place in pot of hot water for about 10 minutes. Drink the tea; then, apply ginger bag to sore area for about a half hour.
- Chop up 1 garlic clove and take like a pill every couple hours.
- Green tea with raw honey & cinnamon 2 to 3 times a day.
- Medical marijuana/cannabis products.
- Drink 20 ounces of water with 1 teaspoon of grated ginger and/or turmeric root, juice of a lemon and pinch of cayenne pepper powder.

Herbs for Inflammation

Bilberry, blessed thistle, boswellia, cat's claw, cayenne, chamomile, clove, devil's claw, fenugreek, feverfew, garlic, ginger, goldenseal, green tea, hibiscus, holy basil, licorice root, malva, mullein, mustard seeds, pau d'arco, prickly ash, rosemary, saffron, skullcap, St. John's wort, tamarind, turmeric, white willow bark and yucca.

Herbs for Pain

Blue vervain, boswellia, butterbur, cat's claw, cayenne, curcumin, devil's claw, feverfew, ginger, holy basil, kava kava, neem, nutmeg, rosemary, Thai kratom, turmeric and white willow bark.

- Thai kratom has a unique blend of alkaloids known to reduce pain. Mix ¼ to ½ teaspoon powder in juice, water, applesauce, herbal tea or use in pill supplement. Make a cup of tea with 1 teaspoon of Thai kratom powder, infuse for 4 hours in room temperature water, keep in refrigerator and drink ¼ cup 4 times a day.
- Turmeric has anti-inflammatory properties and a natural pain reliever.
- White willow bark contains salicin, which acts as an anti-inflammatory that is similar to aspirin.

My Favorite Herbal Combination for Inflammation & Pain
Butterbur, cayenne, devils claw, feverfew, turmeric & white willow bark.

Herbs to Relax Muscles
Black cohosh, blue vervain, catnip, chamomile, lavender, lobelia, kava kava, macafem, peppermint, Thai kratom, valerian and wood betony.

Herbs for Bone Health
Arjuna bark, bamboo, boneset, comfrey, dandelion, goldenrod, horsetail, oat straw, red clover, teasel root and white oak bark.

Take herbs in powdered, tincture, capsule or tea form - use any combination.

My Favorite Combination for Arthritis
Boswellia, devil's claw, comfrey, glucosamine, turmeric, white oak bark & yucca. Encapsulate or mix 1 teaspoon powder combination in juice or water.

Herbal Inflammation Tea Combination

- Chamomile Flower
- Cinnamon Stick
- Green Tea Leaf
- Holy Basil Leaf
- Rosemary Leaf
- Slice Ginger Root
- Slice Horseradish Root
- Hot Pepper
- Slice Turmeric Root
- Slice Yucca Root

Use all above ingredients or any above fresh or dried herbal combination.

Chop up ingredients and simmer 1 cup of ingredients in gallon of water for 30 minutes and strain. Drink 1 cup of cold, warm or hot tea 1 to 3 times a day. Keep tea in refrigerator up to 2 weeks.

Compress - moisten cloth with herbal tea and apply for about 20 to 40 minutes:
- Herb suggestions include cayenne, chamomile, comfrey, feverfew, garlic, ginger root, horseradish root, rosemary, turmeric, white willow bark or yarrow.

Poultice - put fresh or dried herbs in muslin bag or press m' brew tea bags, moisten and apply for about 20 to 40 minutes:
- Herb suggestions include cayenne, chamomile, comfrey, feverfew, garlic, ginger root, horseradish root, rosemary, turmeric, white willow bark or yarrow.

Some Causes of Inflammation

- Dehydration & malnutrition.
- High sugar diet, such as a lot of white sugar, artificial sugar, high fructose corn syrup and all kinds of soda, sports drinks, energy drinks or alcohol. High blood sugar levels suppress the immune system and contributes to the inflammation of muscles, tendons, cartilage and nerves.
- Limit or eliminate bad carbohydrates as much as possible, such as white flour products, pastas, breads, cakes, pies, donuts, french fries or chips.
- Hydrogenated oils or trans fatty acids such as meat drippings, chicken skin, margarine, lard, microwave popcorn or store bought frosting.
- Chemical household and personal products, such as weed and bug poisons, cleaning supplies, detergents, toothpastes, deodorants or air fresheners.
- Excessive red meat and dairy product consumption.
- Food additives, such as preservatives, flavor enhancers, stabilizers or dyes.
- Chronic fungal and viral infections.
- Allergies and heavy metal accumulation.
- Caffeine and carbonation are known to leach calcium and minerals from the bones.
- Cigarette smoking has been known to damage joints, breakdown cartilage and cause damage to nerves and blood vessels which worsen the pain and inflammation.
- Sleeping on arm(s) or have arms(s) over your head while sleeping can cut off circulation.

KARING for KIDNEYS

The kidneys are a pair of kidney bean shaped organs located opposite each other on either side of the spine in back of the abdomen under the diaphragm. Each kidney is about the size of your fist. They remove waste products from the body, produce urine and help maintain fluid balance within the body.

The urinary system consists of the kidneys, bladder, ureters and urethra. It is the plumbing system which stores and then eliminates urine. Caring for the kidneys is known to benefit the whole urinary system and adrenal glands, which are located just above the kidneys.

General Symptoms that the Kidneys Need Attention
- Lines on corners of eyes.
- Ear noise or ringing in the ear.
- Pain in mid to lower back.
- When kidneys fail to properly process fluid, swelling can occur. Can cause ankles, feet, legs, hands, face to swell or puffy eyes.
- Sweaty feet and hands.
- Prone to get morning sickness
- Muscle weakness or twitching.
- Ears and/or hips not level and toes can point inward.
- Bald spots or thinning hair at the widow's peak.
- Phobias, paranoia, panic attacks, insomnia or seizures.
- Barely urinating or urinating frequently. Urine can be foamy, bubbly, cloudy, strong odor, blood streaked and/or a dark color
- Metallic taste in mouth or breath smells of ammonia from buildup of waste.
- Loss of appetite, nausea or food may taste different.
- Pitting edema is when an indent is left in the skin after pushing on skin with fingers.
- When blood vessels in the kidneys get damaged, they cannot filter waste from the blood properly, which can make blood pressure hard to control.
- Kidney stones.

Natural Suggestions to Improve Kidney Health
- Physical activity - 3 times a week or more. Suggestions are walking, biking, gardening, swimming, dancing, stretching, yoga, tai chi or qigong.
- Take breaks from sitting at work and from driving to get circulation going.

- Use a good cushion in the car when driving to block vibration to kidneys.
- Don't suppress your need to urinate. When you need to urinate or have bowel movement, GO as soon as possible!
- Switch to natural household and personal care products or make your own DIY products.
- Compress - warmed castor oil, mustard seed oil or sole water - soak a cotton, muslin or flannel cloth and place over middle of back over kidneys (not on an open wound). Can cover with plastic wrap or a towel and put heating pad or hot water bottle on top; leave on for 30 to 60 minutes. Helps with pain and inflammation.
- Colon hydrotherapy or colonics.
- Ionic foot baths.
- Infrared LED light therapy - helps increase blood flow to injured tissues to help with acne, stretch marks, wrinkles, cellulite, excess pigment, scar tissue, sore muscles and organs.
- Stones & crystals - aquamarine, carnelian, citrine, jade or moonstone. Carry with you or on you, as jewelry, in your pocket, in your purse or lie down with stones on middle of back on each side of spine.
- Essential oils & reflexology to benefit the kidneys - bergamot, chamomile, fennel, grapefruit, helichrysum, juniper, lemon or orange. Choose your own blend and use in a spray, diffuser, car diffuser, bath salts, body oil, massage oil or lotion. Make a warm compress by soaking a cloth in very warm water with 10 to 20 drops and place over middle of back over kidneys; cover with a towel. Mix 3 to 10 drops in 1 to 3 tablespoons any carrier oil & massage middle of back and lower abdomen. Massage arch of feet or massage arch of feet with foot roller or ball.

Internally
- Eat healthier - eat lots of vegetables and fruit; avoid excess animal protein, sugar and carbs.
- Drink plenty of water - drink 50 to 70 % of your body weight in ounces of water daily; water works naturally to flush kidneys of toxins.
- Whole food blender drink daily - ingredient suggestions are asparagus, beet, black radish, corn silk, cordycep, cranberry, cranberry juice, cucumber, cabbage, dandelion leaf, ginger, holy basil leaf, juniper berry, kale, parsley leaf, pumpkin seed and spinach.
- Use a good mineral filled sea salt instead of white table salt.
- Omega fatty acids.
- Sea vegetables such as alaria, arame, bladderwrack, chlorella, nori, dulse, ecklonia cava, Irish moss, kelp, kombu, spirulina & wakame (can eat, powder form or supplement products).

- Mushroom supplement products or tea.
- Black radish supplement.
- Celery seed extract/tincture.
- Cranberry or black cherry concentrate - take 1 tablespoon 3 times a day.
- Pumpkin seed oil or extract.
- Corn silk or cranberry pill supplements.
- Raw kidney glandular pill supplement.
- Watermelon Cleanse, *Essiac Tea* or *Master Cleanse* (see Colon/Cleanses).
- Strive to balance your blood sugar levels (see Blood Sugar Imbalance).

Drink 1 to 3 times a day:
- Glass of unsweetened cranberry or black cherry juice.
- Lemon water (see Lemon Water).
- Apple cider vinegar drink - mix 1 tablespoon apple cider vinegar and 1 tablespoon raw honey in glass of warm water.
- ¼ teaspoon baking soda, 1 tablespoon apple cider vinegar and ¼ teaspoon sea salt in glass of water.

Herbal Help
- Powdered greens (see Powdered Greens).
- Capsule of cayenne or ¼ teaspoon added to glass of water with each meal.
- Digestive bitters.
- Yellow dock root decoction (see Herbs/Tea).

Herbs to Benefit Kidneys
Alcachofa, barberry, basil, bearberry, blessed thistle, blue violet, borage, buchu, cats claw, celery root and seeds, chanca piedra, cleaver, corn silk, couch grass, cramp bark, dandelion root, eclipta prostate, eleuthero, ginger, goldenrod, gravel root, horsetail, juniper berry, marshmallow root, milk thistle, nettle, oat grass, olive leaf, Oregon grape, parsley, red clover, red raspberry leaf, rehmannia, schizandra, sheep sorrel, stone root, queen of the meadow, usnea, uva ursi, turmeric, watermelon seed, white oak bark, wood betony and yellow dock root.

My Favorite Herbal Kidney Combination
Dandelion, juniper berry, parsley, uva ursi & queen of the meadow.

My Favorite Herbal Bladder Combination
Bearberry, cleavers, corn silk, horsetail, juniper berry & white oak bark.

My Favorite Herbal Adrenal Combination
Ashwagandha, Korean ginseng, licorice root, rhodiola & schizandra

Take herbs in powdered, tincture, capsule or tea form; any combination.

Dried Herbal Kidney Tea Combination
- Alfalfa Leaf
- Bearberry Leaf
- Dandelion Leaf or Root
- Green Stevia Leaf
- Juniper Berry
- Horsetail
- Licorice Root
- Nettle Leaf
- Oat Grass
- Parsley Leaf or Root

Use all above ingredients or any above dried herbal combination.

Mix ingredients together and store in closed container. 1 tablespoon dried herbal combination in small press n' brew empty tea bags, tea ball or mesh strainer per cup of boiling water. Steep for 15 to 30 minutes and drink 1 to 3 cups a day.

Fresh Herbal Kidney Tea Combination
- Basil Leaf
- Corn Silk
- Parsley Leaf
- Slice Ginger Root

Chop up above ingredients. Combine and use 1 teaspoon to 1 tablespoon chopped herbs in tea ball or mesh strainer in cup of boiling water. Steep for 15 to 30 minutes and drink 1 to 3 cups a day.

Fresh Seed & Berry Tea Combination
- Celery Seed
- Juniper Berry
- Pumpkin Seed
- Watermelon Seed

Chop or grind up 1 tablespoon of each above ingredients and cover bottom of a pint jar or use a tea ball. Fill jar with boiling water, steep for about 1 hour, strain or remove tea ball and drink tea throughout day.

Some Causes & What Makes it Worse
- Chronic dehydration.
- High sugar diet, such as a lot of white sugar, artificial sugar, high fructose corn syrup and all kinds of sports drinks, energy drinks or alcohol.
- Soda or carbonated beverages may contain high concentration of caffeine, sugar or artificial sugar. Dark sodas, except for root beer, contain a lot of

phosphoric acid, a food additive which dissolves calcium contributing to bone loss and dental erosion.

- Limit or eliminate bad carbohydrates as much as possible, such as white flour products, pastas, breads, cakes, pies, donuts, french fries or chips.
- Hydrogenated oils or trans fatty acids such as meat drippings, chicken skin, margarine, lard, microwave popcorn or store bought frosting.
- Chemical, synthetic household and personal products, such as weed and bug poisons, cleaning supplies, detergents, soaps, air fresheners, make-up, perfumes or dyes.
- Drugs overwork the kidneys, such as antibiotics, diuretics, acetaminophen, aspirin, ibuprofen, any pain medication, synthetic vitamins and much more.
- Limit caffeine which acts as a diuretic and can deter the kidneys absorption of water.
- Cigarette smoking reduces blood flow to the kidneys and damages arteries.
- Excessive use of over-the-counter antacids.
- Heavy metal accumulation.
- Urinary tract or bladder infection.
- Bad sunburns can dehydrate and impact the kidneys.

LOVE YOUR LIVER

The liver is the largest solid organ in the body and is also considered a gland. It's located in the upper right part of the abdomen protected by the ribcage. It has many functions, probably its main job is to filter the blood. The liver also helps break down fat, produces cholesterol, metabolizes drugs and so much more. Caring for the liver is known to benefit the gallbladder, which is located just below the liver.

General Symptoms that the Liver Needs Attention
- Pain between shoulder blades and in middle of the back especially on right side under ribs.
- Swelling of legs and/or swelling beneath the ribs on right side.
- Dark circles under eyes and/or vertical lines between eyebrows.
- Loss of appetite that leads to weight loss, anemia or muscle wasting. The body can become weak with vomiting, diarrhea and nausea.
- Feeling tired a lot and unrefreshed upon waking.
- Jaundice or pale, pasty, yellowish complexion is when color of skin and whites of eyes turn yellow or pale orange.
- Fingernails are whitish or have horizontal ridges.
- Stools become pale and lighter in color, grey or whitish, which is a sign of low bile production.
- Urine can become dark like ice tea.
- Bloody, black and/or tarry stools.
- Bruise and bleed easily (e.g., nose bleeds) - if liver is unable to produce proteins necessary for the blood to clot properly.
- If toxins can't be eliminated from the liver, they will come out of skin. Can lead to skin issues including acne, eczema and rashes.
- Redness in the palms of your hands, chest and face.
- Bad breath, nausea, digestive problems and constipation.
- Sudden seizures, tinnitus and dizziness.
- Bald spot or thinning on top of head.
- Patches of dark skin on neck and underarms.
- Hormonal imbalances such as loss of body hair, increased breast size, decreased testicular size and hot flashes.
- Ingrown toenail on big toe(s).
- Intolerance to drinking alcohol, can get drunk quickly or have unexpected bad hangovers in comparison to what you drank.
- Loss of flexibility of tendon and ligaments.

- Pitting edema is when an indent is left in the skin after pushing on skin with fingers.
- Anemia, cirrhosis, hepatitis, enlarged liver or spleen.

Natural Suggestions to Improve Liver Health
- Physical activity - 3 times a week or more. Suggestions are walking, biking, gardening, swimming, light hand weights, dancing, stretching, yoga, tai chi or qigong. Physical activity helps lower triglycerides and reduce buildup of fat in the liver.
- Switch to natural household and personal care products or make your own DIY products.
- Organic coffee or garlic enema is known to promote the liver to release bile and toxins.
- Colon hydrotherapy or colonics.
- Ionic foot baths.
- Compress - warmed castor oil, mustard seed oil or warm sole water - soak a cotton, muslin or flannel cloth and place on right abdomen over ribs where liver is located (not on open wound). Can cover with plastic wrap or a towel and put heating pad or hot water bottle on top; leave on for 30 to 60 minutes. Helps with pain and inflammation.
- Infrared LED light therapy - helps increase blood flow to injured tissues to help with acne, stretch marks, wrinkles, cellulite, excess pigment, scar tissue, sore muscles and organs.
- Stones & crystals - amber, citrine, aquamarine, red jasper, tiger's eye or topaz. Carry with you or on you, as jewelry, in your pocket, in your purse or lie down with stone on right abdomen over ribs where liver is located.
- Essential oils & reflexology to benefit the liver - black pepper, cedarwood, chamomile, cinnamon, clove, grapefruit, juniper, rosemary, peppermint or thyme. Choose your own blend and use in a spray, diffuser, car diffuser, bath salts, body oil or massage oil or lotion. Make a warm compress, by soaking a cloth in very warm water with 10 to 20 drops, place where liver is located; cover with a towel. Mix 3 to 10 drops in 1 to 3 tablespoons any carrier oil & massage where liver is located. Also, massage arch of feet or massage arch of feet using foot roller or ball.

Internally
- Eat healthier & drink plenty of water.
- Whole food blender drink daily - ingredient suggestions are beet, black radish, burdock root, cabbage, cordycep, cucumber, dandelion leaf & root, kale, parsley leaf, reishi mushroom, spinach, and swiss chard.

- Use a good mineral filled sea salt instead of white table salt.
- About 30% of our daily food intake should be fiber foods. Fiber suggestions include apple pectin, barley, beans, chia seeds, farro, flaxseed meal, hemp hearts, konjac root, lentils nuts, seeds, oats, peas, psyllium husks, sprouted breads, quinoa, fruits and vegetables.
- Apple cider vinegar drink - 1 tablespoon each of apple cider vinegar and raw honey in glass of warm water; stir and drink 1 to 3 times a day.
- Garlic - swallow 1 to 3 chopped cloves like a pill, as a tincture, tea or pill supplement.
- Black radish supplement.
- Sea vegetables such as alaria, arame, bladderwrack, chlorella, nori, dulse, ecklonia cava, Irish moss, kelp, kombu, spirulina & wakame (can eat, powder form or supplement products).
- Omega fatty acids.
- Mushroom supplement products or tea.
- Kombucha mushroom tea; buy or make.
- Raw liver glandular pill supplement.
- Detox vegetable tea - produce suggestions include burdock leaf, cabbage leaf, cilantro leaf, collard green, dandelion green, fennel leaf, garlic clove, ginger root, horseradish root, kale leaf, leek, mustard green, onion, parsley leaf & turnip green. Simmer in gallon of water as many ingredients that you have available for about 30 minutes. Strain and drink cup of warm or cold tea 2 to 4 times a day. Keep in refrigerator for up to 1 week.
- Tamarind tea detox - bring 6 cups of water with 5 to 10 cut in half tamarind pods to a boil and simmer for 30 minutes. Remove pods and drink ½ cup of hot, room temperature or cold tea 2 to 4 times a day. Keep in refrigerator for up to 1 week.
- Watermelon Cleanse, *Essiac Tea* or *Master Cleanse* (see Colon/Cleanses).
- Strive to balance your blood sugar levels (see Blood Sugar Imbalance).

Herbal Help
- Powdered greens (see Powdered Greens).
- Milk thistle pill supplement, apple cider vinegar tincture; buy or make or add 1 teaspoon of milk thistle powder to powdered greens or whole food blender drink.
- Yellow dock root decoction (see Herbs/Tea).
- Digestive bitters.
- Chaparral, dandelion, wormwood and/or pau d'arco tea cleanse - use fresh or dried herbs; fill pint jar ¼ full of herb(s), fill with hot water, let sit for hour and drink 1 pint a day for 2 weeks.

Herbs to Benefit Liver
Alcachofa, barberry, bhringraj, black root, blessed thistle, blue vervain, blue violet, borututu bark, bupleurum, burdock root, clementine, chanca piedra, chaparral, chicory root, comfrey, dandelion, echinacea, eclipta prostrata, gentian root, goldenseal, kudzu, licorice root, milk thistle, nettle, oat grass, olive leaf, Oregon grape, nigella sativa, oldenlandia diffusa, parsley, pau d'arco, prickly ash bark, psoralea corylifolia fruit, red clover, rehmannia, rhubarb root, sarsaparilla, schizandra, turmeric and yellow dock root

My Favorite Herbal Liver Combination
Barberry, dandelion, milk thistle, olive leaf, Oregon grape & turmeric

Take herbs in powdered, tincture, capsule or tea form - use any combination.

Dried Herbal Love Your Liver Tea Combination

• Alcachofa Leaf	• Milk Thistle Seed
• Chaparral Leaf	• Olive Leaf
• Burdock Root	• Parsley Leaf
• Dandelion Leaf or Root	• Pau D'arco Bark
• Juniper Berry	• Yellow Dock Root

Use all above ingredients or any above dried herbal combination.

Mix ingredients together and store in closed container. 1 tablespoon dried herbal combination in small press n' brew empty tea bags, tea ball or mesh strainer per cup of boiling water. Steep for 15 to 30 minutes and drink 1 to 3 cups a day.

Some Causes & What Makes it Worse
- High sugar diet, such as lot of white sugar, artificial sugar, high fructose corn syrup and all kinds of soda, sports drinks or energy drinks.
- Excessive alcohol consumption.
- Limit or eliminate bad carbohydrates as much as possible, such as white flour products, pastas, breads, cakes, pies, donuts, french fries or chips.
- Foods containing high sodium or MSG (monosodium glutamate), such as deli meats, soy sauce, fast food, chips, microwave dinners or sausages.
- Hydrogenated oils or trans fatty acids, such as meat drippings, chicken skin, margarine, lard, microwave popcorn or store bought frosting.
- Chemical household and personal products, such as weed and bug poisons, cleaning supplies, detergents, toothpastes, deodorants or air fresheners.

- Drugs overwork the liver, such as antibiotics, diuretics, acetaminophen, aspirin, ibuprofen, any pain medication, synthetic vitamins and much more.
- Heavy metal accumulation.

REMEDIES FOR COMMON AILMENTS & FIRST AID

Acne

Some common causes include dehydration, hormone imbalance, sluggish liver, stress & anxiety.

- Ground inner leaves of cabbage - lie down, apply to blemishes. Leave on about 15 to 30 minutes; rinse off with warm water.
- Facial clay mask - mix together 2 tablespoons of clay such as bentonite clay, french green clay or kaolin clay, 1 tablespoon activated charcoal powder with 2 to 5 tablespoons apple cider vinegar. Apply to face and neck, leave on about 15 minutes; rinse off with warm water. Use daily for 1 to 2 weeks and then once a week as maintenance for stubborn acne.
- Infrared LED light therapy helps increase blood flow to injured tissues to help with acne, stretch marks, wrinkles, cellulite, excess pigment, scar tissue, sore muscles and organs.
- Yellow dock root tea - make & drink tea. Put warm softened roots in small press n' brew empty tea bag or tie in small piece of cloth, or moisten cotton ball with tea and apply to blemish for 15 to 30 minutes.
- Rosewater & lemon toner - 2 tablespoons rosewater and juice of half lemon, apply to face and neck. Leave on about 15 to 30 minutes; rinse off with warm water.
- Facial steam - fill a large bowl half full with boiling water & aloe vera leaf, fresh or dried basil leaves, chamomile flowers, lavender flowers, oregano leaves, rose petals, few drops each of lavender & tea tree essential oils. Use all ingredients or whatever you have available. With a towel over head, bend over bowl for about 5 to 15 minutes.
- Acne, scars and stretch marks - mix 1 to 3 drops of frankincense, lavender and/or chamomile essential oils with 3 to 5 drops of vitamin E oil; massage into area daily.

Apply a few times a day with fingertip, gauze pad or q-tip:
- Slice of garlic clove or Garlic Oil (see DIY Recipes).
- Hazel Toner (see DIY Recipes).
- Witch hazel.
- Sole water (see Himalayan Sea Salt).
- Sanitizing Oil (see DIY Recipes).

- Colloidal silver.
- Undiluted tea tree essential oil.
- Aloe vera gel scraped from leaf.
- Piece of inside of banana peel.
- Raw honey.
- Apple cider vinegar.
- Juice of half lemon.
- Bruised moist basil leaves.
- Cucumber seed oil.
- Bentonite clay & tea tree oil.
- Turmeric powder & colloidal silver.
- Baking soda & honey.
- Whiteheads - wet cotton ball with sole water, put on whitehead for about 20 minutes, then follow with dab of honey or tea tree essential oil.
- Essential oils such as clary sage, frankincense, lavender, oregano, rosemary or tea tree. Mix 3 to 10 drops of essential oils of your choice in 1 tablespoon of jojoba oil or carrier oil of your choice.

Internally
- Eat healthier & drink plenty of water.
- Activated charcoal products.
- Helps many people to balance hormones (see Hormone Imbalance).
- Herbs to strengthen the liver are known to help (see Love Your Liver); if toxins can't be eliminated from the liver, they will come out of skin.

Allergies & Colds

Raising our immune system strengthens our body to be better equipped in fighting off infections.

- Physical activity gets the blood moving which help raises our immune system - 3 times a week or more. Suggestions are walking, biking, yoga, gardening, swimming, dancing, tai chi or qigong.
- Neti pot or bulb syringe - up of warm water mixed with a ½ teaspoon of sea salt or sole water and ½ teaspoon of colloidal silver; bend over sink or bowl, tilt head to one side and pour half into one nostril until liquid comes out other nostril into sink; then do other side.
- Salt blend used in neti pot can also be used as a nasal spray.
- Nasal hygiene systems.
- Himalayan sea salt inhaler.
- Wild yam ginger spray.
- Steam inhalers - optional to add 1 tablespoon of colloidal silver to water.

- Oil pulling draws out toxins and bacteria by swishing 1 tablespoon of sesame seed oil or coconut oil back and forth, front and back through teeth for 5 to 20 minutes; then spit out and rinse.
- Slice up white or red onions, place on bottom of feet and keep in place by putting on a pair socks to act as an antibiotic, helps detox toxins and increases hydration.
- For a cold, place bowls of cut up onions near you while you sleep to absorb bacteria and toxins. Throw out after 24 hours and replenish as needed.
- Ginger compress - 1 tablespoon grated ginger in cup of hot water, steep washcloth in ginger water for 5 minutes and squeeze out water. Lie down, close eyes and place warm moist towel over face and breathe.
- Cinnamon paste - mix a little water with 1 teaspoon of cinnamon powder and apply paste to nose and forehead to help clear nasal passages.
- Buy or make menthol salve or oil - rub on chest and upper back for decongestion and under your nose, in your nose and facial sinus areas to open up sinuses.
- Facial steam - fill a large bowl half full with boiling water & ¼ cup apple cider vinegar, fresh or dried peppermint leaves, eucalyptus leaves, slice of ginger root, aloe vera leaf, sliced garlic clove, few whole cloves, few drops each of ravansara & thyme essential oils. Use all ingredients or whatever you have available. With a towel over head, bend over bowl; breath for about 5 to 15 minutes.
- Use gua sha tools on neck, chest, shoulders and upper back.
- Essential oils & reflexology to fight infections - black pepper, cedarwood, cinnamon, clove, eucalyptus, frankincense, ginger, marjoram, mullein, oregano, peppermint, pine, ravensara, rosemary, sandalwood, spruce, tea tree or thyme. Choose your own blend and use in diffuser, spray, facial steam, humidifier or vaporizer. Mix 3 to 10 drops in 1 to 3 tablespoons any carrier oil & massage neck, chest, upper back and belly. Massage both feet for five minutes each.

Bath - add one of following in warm to hot bath water and soak for about 15 to 30 minutes; suggestion to shower after to rinse off toxins:
- ½ cup to 1 cup apple cider vinegar, bentonite clay, sea salt or sole water or any combination.
- Bath bag - mix together crushed cinnamon sticks, slice ginger root, sea salt and eucalyptus leaves. Put mixed blend into large press n' brew empty tea bags, muslin bags, old sock tied closed or large tea ball.
- ½ cup to 1 cup Bath Powder Blend (see DIY Recipes).
- Foot baths - 2 tablespoons to ½ cup of any suggestion above.

Internally
- Eat healthier & drink plenty of water.
- Whole food blender drink daily - ingredients suggestions are acai berry, aloe vera leaf, bee pollen, carrot, cinnamon stick, collard green, colostrum powder, elderberry, garlic, ginger, goji berry, grapefruit, horseradish, kale, lemon, mushrooms, onion, peppermint leaf and spinach.
- Powdered greens (see Powdered Greens).
- Bentonite clay water or pill supplement helps remove allergens and toxins.
- Drink lemon water first thing in morning on an empty stomach.
- Grate 1 tablespoon of horseradish root or 2 sliced garlic cloves and place between teeth and gums. Hold for about twenty minutes and spit out. Helps loosen up mucus.
- Elderberry tea, lozenges, capsules or tincture.
- Onions are an expectorant. Soak sliced onions and peeled garlic in raw honey overnight; take 1 tablespoon of infused honey a few times a day.
- Bone broth, gelatin or collagen powder - best to look for grass-fed, pasture raised or organic.
- Eat homemade bone broth chicken soup with garlic and lots of onion.
- Possible vitamins A, C and/or D deficiency (see Minerals/Vitamins).
- Amla berry or camu camu herbal pill supplement.
- Cod liver oil or pill supplement.
- Mushroom supplement products or tea.
- Oregano essential oil pill supplement.
- Some homeopathic and natural cold remedy products online are *Calm Cold, Cold Eeze, Cold Snap, Cold Atak, Oscillococcinum, Zicam* or *Las Vegas Allergy Mix* (for people living in the southwest).

Take daily to strengthen and raise immune system or 3 to 6 times a day when a cold, infection or allergy is present:
- Infection Fighter Herbal Tincture (see DIY Recipes).
- Super Tonic (see DIY Recipes).
- Apple cider vinegar drink - mix 1 tablespoon apple cider vinegar and 1 tablespoon raw honey in glass of warm water.
- Apple cider vinegar shot - in shot glass, 1 tablespoon apple cider vinegar, 1 teaspoon of raw honey and squeeze in juice of half lemon.
- Garlic-lemon shot - in shot glass, squeeze juice of half lemon and 1 crushed garlic clove; fill with water and drink right away.
- Garlic - cut up 1 to 3 cloves and swallow like a pill, as a tincture, tea or pill supplement.
- Cut up slice of horseradish root and swallow like a pill.

- Super fruit juices including acai, goji, mangosteen, noni or pomegranate.
- Bee pollen benefits intestinal flora to strengthen immune system.
- Colloidal silver.
- Grapefruit seed extract products.
- Echinacea and/or goldenseal tincture.
- Colostrum products - colostrum is the first milky fluid your breasts produce in late pregnancy and in the first few breastfeeding days after giving birth. It provides nutrition and stimulates the growth of normal gut organisms that are important for digestive system and raises immune system.

Herbal Help

- Honey gel tea - fill glass jar with 3 parts sliced lemons and 1 part sliced ginger root; then fill with raw honey. Cover and put jar into the refrigerator; it will turn into a gel. Make tea with 1 tablespoon of gel in cup of hot water. Could last about 3 months in the refrigerator.
- Combo tea - combine 1 tablespoon raw honey, ¼ to ½ teaspoon cinnamon powder, juice of half lemon, 2 slices of ginger root and dash of cayenne powder in a cup of hot water or green tea; drink 2 to 3 times a day.

Infection Fighting and Strengthen Immune System Herbs (have antibiotic, antibacterial and/or antiviral properties to fight viral & bacterial infections)
Acacia, acerola, aloe vera, amla berry, ashwagandha, astragalus, boneset, blue violet, camu camu, cats claw, chamomile, chaparral, cinnamon, comfrey, echinacea, elderberry, elderflower, garlic, ginger, goldenseal, hibiscus, holy basil, horseradish, juniper, lemon balm, licorice root, moringa, myrrh, olive leaf, oregano, Oregon grape, osha root, red root, roschip, sage, star anise, tamarind, Thai kratom, thyme, turmeric, usnea, white willow bark, wild indigo, wormwood and yarrow

Expectorant Herbs (to help get rid of mucus & chest congestion)
Black cumin seeds, brigham tea, chaparral, coltsfoot, elecampane root, eucalyptus, fennel, fenugreek, horehound, horseradish, hyssop, lobelia, lungwort, malva, marshmallow root, mullein, nettle, oregano, peppermint, red clover, thyme, umckaloabo and wild cherry bark

Decongestant Herbs (to help clear a stuffy nose)
Astragalus, black cumin seeds, brigham tea, cayenne, chamomile, cinnamon, curry leaves, echinacea, ephedra, eucalyptus, eyebright, garlic, ginger, green tea, horseradish, licorice root, lobelia, mullein, osha, peppermint, sage, thyme and umckaloabo

Antihistamine Herbs (to help with sneezing, runny nose, itching)
Basil, butterbur, chamomile, echinacea, elderberry, eyebright, fennel, garlic, ginger, goldenrod, goldenseal, green tea, horny goat weed, licorice root, nettle, papaya, peppermint, reishi mushroom and thyme.

My Favorite Infection Fighting & Raise Immune System Herbal Combination
Astragalus, echinacea, elderberry, myrrh & yarrow.

Take herbs in powder, tincture, capsule or tea form - use any combination.

My Favorite Allergy Combination (clay & powdered herbs)
Bentonite clay, butterbur, echinacea, eyebright, ginger, horehound, mullein & nettle. Encapsulate or mix 1 teaspoon of powder combination in juice or water.

Herbal Infection Fighting & Immune System Tea Combination
- Amla Berry
- Chamomile Flower
- Echinacea Leaf or Root
- Elderberry
- Eucalyptus Leaf
- Ginger Root
- Holy Basil Leaf
- Horseradish Root
- Licorice Root
- Mullein Leaf
- Peppermint Leaf
- Turmeric Root

Use all above ingredients or any above fresh or dried herbal combination.

Chop up ingredients and simmer 1 cup of ingredients in gallon of water for about 30 minutes and strain. Drink 1 cup of cold, warm or hot tea 1 to 3 times a day. Keep tea in refrigerator up to 2 weeks.

At the first sign of a cold or infection, it is important to strengthen the immune system - I will take Infection Fighter Herbal Tincture (see DIY Recipes) or Super Tonic (see DIY Recipes). Take 3 squirts or 1 teaspoon every hour the first day and every two hours the second day. Then, every 3 to 5 hours for a week or until I feel better. Feel free to combine with above remedies including teas, gargles, baths and staying hydrated.

Bleeding
- Warm sea salt water - 1 teaspoon of sea salt, stir into ½ cup of warm water; or pour sole water over area and then apply pressure.
- Place moistened green or black tea bag on wound or extracted tooth to stop bleeding and help blood to clot.
- Ice cube on affected area for about 30 seconds.

Apply to cut or wound:
- Cayenne or turmeric powder.
- Crushed yarrow leaves or powder.
- Raw honey.
- Apple cider vinegar or witch hazel on a cotton ball.
- Juniper tree sap.

Nose Bleed:
- Pinch nose and bend forward with your head between your legs.
- Pinch of cayenne in nostril.
- Sniff a sliced onion.
- Hold ice cube on roof of mouth as long as you can or until bleeding stops.
- Moisten a cotton ball with apple cider vinegar and place in nostril.

Burns

1st degree: skin is unbroken; 2nd degree: skin is blistered and/or broken. These ideas are to help minor burns. Seek medical help for moderate & severe burns.
Apply to burned area:
- Cold running water immediately after burning.
- Moistened green or black tea bags.
- Potatoes slices.
- Cucumber slices.
- Mashed cabbage leaves poultice.
- Grated carrot poultice.
- Fresh bruised herb leaves such as chickweed, comfrey, mullein or plantain.
- Cool herbal tea compress - moisten cloth with cooled herbal tea - herb suggestions include chickweed, comfrey, mullein, lavender flowers, plantain, slippery elm or St. John's Wort.
- Poultice - put fresh, powdered or dried herbs in press n' brew empty tea bag or muslin bag, moisten and apply. Herb suggestions include chickweed, comfrey, mullein, lavender flowers, plantain, slippery elm or St. John's Wort.

Apply a few times a day with fingertip, gauze pad or q-tip:
- Aloe vera gel scraped from leaf - soothes inflammation while stimulating collagen and skin regeneration or *Aloe Life Skin Gel*.
- Apple cider vinegar and/or extra virgin olive oil.
- Lavender herbal oil.
- Raw honey.

- Vitamin E oil.
- Wheat germ oil.
- Witch hazel.
- Yellow mustard.
- Straight lavender or tea tree essential oil.
- Mix aloe gel and/or raw honey with lavender and/or tea tree essential oil
- Buy or make burn herbal oil or salve using herbs such as aloe vera powder, comfrey, calendula and/or lavender and essential oils like davana, lavender and/or tea tree (see Herb/Oil/Salves).
- Hazel Toner (see DIY Recipes).
- Healing Salve (see DIY Recipes).

Cough

- Rub menthol salve on bottom of feet and put on socks before going to bed and rub on chest, neck and upper back (see DIY Recipes).

Internally

- Make Herbal Cough Syrup or raw honey cough syrups (see DIY Recipes).
- Fresh grated ginger root tea - 1 tablespoon grated ginger into cup of hot water, let steep for about 10 minutes; optional to add lemon juice, raw honey, cinnamon stick, garlic clove, pinch of cayenne or whole clove.
- Put ½ teaspoon sole water on tongue.
- Mix 1 ounce aloe vera juice or gel with 1 teaspoon of mucilage herbs including slippery elm bark powder, coltsfoot powder, marshmallow root powder or mullein powder; drink to soothe and coat esophagus to enhance healing.
- Slippery elm, zinc, horehound or black licorice lozenges.
- Elderberry cough syrup, lozenges or tincture.
- Wild lettuce, coltsfoot, red clover and/or sage tea.
- Chew on slice of licorice root.
- Super Tonic (see DIY Recipes).
- Buy natural cough drops products.

Diarrhea

- Essential oils & reflexology - chamomile, ginger, lavender, peppermint or nutmeg. Mix 3 to 10 drops of essential oils of your choice in 1 to 3 tablespoons any carrier oil of & massage abdomen, both feet and toes.

Internally
- Slippery elm bark powder - stir 1 tablespoon in glass of water; drink after meals and/or at bedtime.
- Add 1 tablespoon slippery elm bark powder to applesauce, yogurt, pudding or kefir.
- Activated charcoal pill supplement.
- 1 tablespoon dry chia seeds.
- Okra tea.
- Oregano essential oil pill supplement.
- Peppermint tea.
- Ginger pill supplement, chew on ginger root or crystallized ginger chews.
- Fresh grated ginger root tea - 1 tablespoon grated ginger into cup of hot water, let steep for about 10 minutes; optional to add lemon juice, raw honey, cinnamon stick, garlic clove, pinch of cayenne or whole clove.
- Cinnamon water - 1 teaspoon cinnamon powder in glass of water.
- Hot cinnamon tea - 1 teaspoon cinnamon powder, few whole cloves and cinnamon stick in cup of hot water.
- Eat a banana or make whole food blender drink containing banana, apples, okra, cinnamon stick and few peppermint leaves.
- Stir 1 teaspoon bentonite clay or food grade diatomaceous earth in water, juice or coconut water. Drink 1 to 3 times a day about a half hour before meals or mix in applesauce, yogurt or pudding.
- Helps to drink glass of water with 1 tablespoon sea salt or sole water and 1 tablespoon raw honey or make Sports/Electrolyte Drink (see DIY Recipes).

Cup of warm whole milk with:
- 1 teaspoon of allspice powder.
- ½ teaspoon each of cinnamon powder & clove powder.
- 1 teaspoon of carob powder.

Digestion Health
Acid reflux & heartburn.

- Avoid caffeine, cigarettes, alcohol, carbonation, refined sugars, antacids, acid blockers, carbohydrates, food preservatives and wearing tight clothing.
- Stabilize weight to be appropriate for your size.
- Raise head 6 to 8 inches while sleeping.
- Eat small, frequent, healthier meals; don't overeat.
- Avoid eating 2 to 3 hours before bedtime.

- Essential oils & reflexology to aid digestion - clove, fennel, ginger, lemon, peppermint, oregano or tangerine. Mix 3 to 10 drops of essential oils of your choice in 1 to 3 tablespoons any carrier oil & massage belly, base of hand where wrist begins and arch area of both feet or use foot roller or ball.

Internally
- Drink lots of water - 2 to 4 quarts a day will help neutralize acids in stomach. A glass of water 30 minutes before a meal can help with digestion.
- Drink lemon water first thing in morning on empty stomach.
- Apple cider vinegar - take 1 tablespoon straight, followed by a glass of water or herbal tea for heartburn attack. Also, take 1 tablespoon apple cider vinegar in glass of water or herbal tea daily.
- Upon waking each morning and before eating or drinking, stir 1 tablespoon sole water in a glass of water.
- Mix and drink 1 teaspoon of baking soda in 4 ounces of water.
- Plant based digestive enzyme pill supplements like papain from papaya and bromelain from pineapple. They may be needed when the body doesn't produce enough enzymes to break down our food.
- Digestive enzyme pill supplements like amylase, lipase and protease.
- Kombucha mushroom tea; buy or make.
- Bone broth, gelatin or collagen powder - best to look for grass-fed, pasture raised or organic.
- Black radish products.
- 1 to 3 tablespoons chia seed gel.
- Almond milk smoothie with banana, pineapple & berries.
- Aloe vera juice or gel - drink 1 or 2 ounces of aloe vera juice before meals.
- Copper infused water - store water for 8 hours or overnight in 100% copper vessel, for instance a pitcher, mug or water bottle and drink 1 to 2 glasses a day for its anti-inflammatory, antibacterial and antiviral properties.
- Eat bitter foods & herbs like arugula, bitter melon, blessed thistle, chicory, dandelion greens, chamomile, dark chocolate, dill, endive, fenugreek seeds, gentian, goldenseal, horseradish, Jerusalem artichoke, kale, lettuce, milk thistle, nettle, parsley, radish, saffron, sesame seeds, turmeric, watercress, wormwood and yarrow.
- Digestive bitters.
- Slippery elm bark powder - stir 1 teaspoon to 1 tablespoon in glass of water; drink after meals and/or at bedtime.

- Add 1 tablespoon slippery elm bark powder to applesauce, yogurt, kefir or pudding.
- Chew on a slice of licorice root or ginger root.
- Ginger pill supplement, chew on ginger root or crystallized ginger chews.
- Fresh grated ginger root tea - 1 tablespoon grated ginger into cup of hot water, let steep for about 10 minutes; optional to add lemon juice, raw honey, cinnamon stick, garlic clove, pinch of cayenne or whole clove.
- Oregano essential oil pill supplement.
- Medical marijuana/cannabis products.
- Peppermint tea.
- Peppermint essential oil pill supplement.
- A drop or two of therapeutic grade peppermint essential oil in cup of water or herbal tea to benefit heartburn and digestion.
- Yellow dock root decoction (see Herbs/Tea).
- Super Tonic (see DIY Recipes).

Herbs to Help with Digestion

Alcachofa leaf, aloe vera, apple pectin, barberry root, black pepper, bladderwrack, blessed thistle, cardamom, caraway, cascara sagrada, catnip, cayenne, chamomile, Chinese goldthread, cinnamon, cumin, dill, duhat, fennel, fenugreek, gentian root, ginger, herba buena, hibiscus, lemon balm, licorice root, marshmallow root, mullein, peppermint, persimmon leaf, psyllium seed, sage, senna, slippery elm bark, star anise, turmeric, white oak bark and wild lettuce

Take herbs in powder, tincture, capsule or tea form - use any combination.

Herbal Digestion & Stomach Tea Combination

- Catnip Leaf
- Chamomile Flower
- Cinnamon Powder or Stick
- Dill Leaf
- Fennel Seed
- Fenugreek Seed
- Peppermint Leaf
- Sage Leaf
- Licorice Root
- Slippery Elm Bark
- Star Anise
- Wild Lettuce Leaf

Use all above ingredients or any above fresh or dried herbs & ground seeds combination.

Chop up ingredients and simmer 1 cup of ingredients in gallon of water for 30 minutes and strain. Mix strained tea with 3 to 5 cups of unsweetened organic apple juice. Drink ½ cup to 1 cup of warm to hot tea after each meal. Keep tea in refrigerator up to 2 weeks.

Ear Infection

- Onion poultice - slice up onion, wrap slices in muslin cloth or bag; apply to outside of ear and squeeze a couple of drops of onion juice in ear(s).
- Ear candling - helps pull out bacteria, loosens wax buildup, helps dry up swimmers ear and relieves some sinus pressure.
- Excess ear wax (sometimes mistaken for an ear infection) - put drop or two of hydrogen peroxide in ear for a minute.

Put a drop or two in ear canal:
- Herbal ear oil with mullein.
- Garlic Oil or tincture.
- Chaparral oil or tincture.
- Apple cider vinegar.
- Colloidal silver.
- Lobelia tincture or oil.

Energy Level
Natural suggestions to boost energy.

- Physical activity - 3 times a week or more. Suggestions are walking, biking, gardening, swimming, dancing, stretching, yoga, tai chi or qigong.
- Headstand or handstand against wall for 1 minute; such inversions can boost energy for 3 hours.
- Deep breathing - breath in slowly through nose for about 5 to 7 seconds; your stomach should expand. Hold breath for about 5 to 7 seconds or longer; then, slowly breathe all of the air out of mouth for about 5 to 10 seconds. Keep repeating. Do this anytime for about 5 to 10 minutes. Deep breathing is relaxing and good for stress, anxiety, adrenals and lungs.
- Get enough sleep - 6 to 9 hours nightly.
- Wear bright colors.

Internally
- Drink plenty of water - at least half your body weight in ounces daily; dehydration can cause fatigue.
- Whole food blender drink 1 or 2 times a day.
- Powdered greens and maybe have another glass in the afternoon for a pick me up.
- Apple cider vinegar drink - 1 tablespoon each of apple cider vinegar and raw honey in glass of warm water; stir and drink 1 to 3 times a day.
- Cordyceps or reishi mushroom products or teas.
- Possible iron and/or vitamin B12 deficiency (see Minerals & Vitamins).

- Bee pollen or royal jelly.
- Omega fatty acids.
- Protein powder drinks.
- Green tea.
- Yerba mate tea.
- Chai drinks.
- Shot of wheatgrass.
- Natural organic energy drinks.
- Glass of grape juice with dash of cayenne.
- Sea vegetables such as alaria, arame, bladderwrack, chlorella, nori, dulse, ecklonia cava, Irish moss, kelp, kombu, spirulina & wakame (can eat, powder form or supplement products).
- Essential oils such as black pepper, cypress, eucalyptus, frankincense, grapefruit, lemon, orange, peppermint or rosemary. Choose your own essential oil blend. Use in a spray, roll-on, eye pillow, diffuser, car diffuser, bath salts, body oil or lotion. Put a few drops on a cotton ball, keep the cotton ball in a plastic bag and smell when needed.

Herbs to Increase Energy

Ashwagandha, Asian ginseng, cayenne, cinnamon, fo-ti, ginger, ginkgo, gotu kola, green tea, guarana seed, kola nut, maca root, ma huang or ephedra, nettle, prickly pear cactus, red panax, rhodiola rosea, schisandra berry, Siberian ginseng, spirulina, turmeric, yerba mate and yellow dock root.

My Favorite Herbal Energy Combination

Green tea, guarana & Siberian ginseng.

Take herbs in powdered, tincture, capsule or tea form.

Eye Health

- Herbal eye wash tea - combine 1 teaspoon eyebright powder, 1 teaspoon of comfrey powder, ½ teaspoon goldenseal powder and pinch of cayenne powder in glass jar. Top off with 1 cup of boiled distilled water; stir and let cool to room temperature and strain; store tea in refrigerator. Use eyecup, dropper or put into a spray bottle. Good for eye issues including allergies, dry eyes or cataracts. Can also make a compress by dipping cloth in tea and placing over closed eyes.
- Eye infection or allergies - 1 drop of echinacea and/or goldenseal tea in eyes a few times a day.
- Bentonite clay poultice - place 1 teaspoon clay in small press n' brew empty tea bag and place on closed eyes.

- Something in eye - put one flaxseed in corner of eye before going to bed, by morning seed should come out on its own with object stuck to it.
- *Miracle II* neutralizer liquid or colloidal silver in spray bottle or dropper bottle for allergies and dry or irritated eyes.

Bags under eyes, puffy eyes or black eye:
- Place cucumber slices or potato slices on closed eyes.
- Moist cooled green tea bag and/or chamomile tea bag or make your own using small press n' brew empty tea bag and place on closed eyes.
- Dampen gauze pad with sole water, rosewater or copper infused water and place on closed eye.

Internally
- Possible vitamin A deficiency (see Minerals & Vitamins).
- Grape seed extract supplement products.
- Drink cup of carrot and fennel juice or blender drink daily.

Herbs to Benefit Eyes
Asphalatus, bilberry, bilway, blackcurrant, coleus forskohlii, comfrey, eyebright, fennel, ginkgo biloba, goldenseal, jaborandi, medical marijuana, passion flower, saffron and triphala

My Favorite Herbal Eye Combination
Bilberry, coleus forskohlii & eyebright

Take herbs in powder, tincture, capsule or tea form - use any combination. These herbs help with night vision, blurry vision, cataracts, near or far sightedness.

Food Poisoning
Ideas for mild poisoning. For moderate to severe cases, seek medical help.
Internally
Take a few times a day till better:
- Activated charcoal products.
- Apple cider vinegar - 1 tablespoon of apple cider vinegar in glass of warm water or herbal tea.
- Mix 2 tablespoons bentonite clay in glass of water; stir and drink.
- Ginger pill supplement, chew on ginger root or crystallized ginger chews.
- Cinnamon water - 1 teaspoon of cinnamon powder in glass of water.
- Hot cinnamon tea - 1 teaspoon of cinnamon powder, few whole cloves and cinnamon stick in cup of hot water.
- Take 1 teaspoon of fresh lemon juice and/or raw honey.

- Peppermint tea.
- Peppermint essential oil pill supplement.
- Mix 1 teaspoon fenugreek or fennel seeds with 3 tablespoons yogurt.
- Burdock root & ginger root tea.
- Colloidal silver.
- Garlic - swallow 1 chopped garlic clove like a pill, or as a tincture, tea or pill supplement. Also helps to rub belly with garlic oil.

Hair Loss

Some causes for hair loss are malnutrition, scalp fungal infection, hormone or thyroid imbalance. Research indicates some medications contribute to hair loss, especially steroids.

Apply one of the following to scalp and leave on for at least 30 minutes before washing hair;
- Castor oil & cayenne pepper powder.
- Aloe vera gel scraped from leaf and coconut milk.
- Cucumber seed oil or bhringraj oil.
- Vitamin E oil mixed with coconut oil.
- Kokum oil & butter, jojoba oil, mango seed oil & butter, mustard seed oil or sapote oil.
- Hyaluronic acid products.
- Rosemary & sage tea.
- Essential oils to stimulate hair growth are birch, clary sage, lavender, peppermint, rosemary, sage or tea tree. Mix 5 to 10 drops of essential oils of your choice in 2 tablespoons of jojoba oil, neem oil, sesame seed oil or mustard seed oil.
- Make herbal hormonal oil, salve or cream. Herb suggestions include black cohosh, chaste tree berries, damiana, red raspberry, sage and wild yam (see Herbs/Oils/Salves).

Internally
- Helps many people to balance hormones (see Hormone Imbalance).
- Possible copper, iodine and/or protein deficiency (see Minerals & Vitamins).
- Whole food blender drink daily - ingredient suggestions are alfalfa, almond, avocado, blackcurrant oil, borage oil, broccoli, cabbage, chaste tree berry, cucumber, evening primrose oil, kale, mustard green, pumpkin seed, quinoa, romaine lettuce, rosemary leaf, sage leaf, sprouts and spinach.
- Spirulina and/or chlorella products.

- Bone broth, gelatin or collagen powder - best to look for grass-fed, pasture raised or organic.
- Cucumber juice; make or buy.
- Copper peptides.
- Copper infused water - store water for 8 hours or overnight in 100% copper vessel, for instance a pitcher, mug or water bottle and drink 1 to 2 glasses a day for its anti-inflammatory, antibacterial and antiviral properties.

Herbs to Promote Hair Growth

Bamboo, bhringraj, ecklonia cava, horsetail, neem, nettle, oat grass, rosemary, sage, sarsaparilla and saw palmetto.

My Favorite Herbal Powder Hair Growth Combination

Bamboo, horsetail, oat grass, rosemary & sage.

Take herbs in powder, tincture, capsule or tea form - use any combination.

Headaches

- Get plenty of sleep (see First Aid/Sleep).
- Avoid caffeine, alcohol and cigarettes.
- Be cautious of chemical household and personal products, such as cleaning supplies, clothes detergents, perfumes and air fresheners.
- EFT or Emotion Freedom Technique - a process of tapping areas of the body to clear out negative energy blockages. Helps with pain, stress, fear, inflammation, depression, anxiety and headaches. EFT is easy to learn and easy to do on yourself.
- Enemas or colon hydrotherapy.
- Use gua sha tools on neck, shoulders and upper back.
- Cefaly is a transcutaneous electrical nerve stimulation (TENS) machine unit for the head.
- Massage therapy to help loosen muscles, increase circulation and relieve tension and stress.
- Acupuncture, chiropractic or reiki.
- Put hands in bowl of ice water for as long as you can take it, while opening and closing fingers into a fist.
- Cold compress or bag of frozen peas on forehead and back of neck.
- Cold sole water compress; moisten cloth and apply with cooled sole water to forehead and back of neck.
- Cold herbal tea compress - make white willow bark and/or feverfew herbal tea; cool in refrigerator. Steep 2 cloths in tea. Place one on forehead

and one on back of neck for about a half hour. Optional at the same time; soak feet in hot foot bath with 2 tablespoons bentonite clay, mustard powder and/or ginger powder.

- Frozen cabbage leaves on forehead and back of neck.
- Herbal headache eye pillow - use half peppermint & eucalyptus leaves with flax seeds; buy or make.
- Menthol Salve or Dit Dat Jow - rub on temples, forehead and back of neck and top of shoulders.
- CBD products.
- Medical marijuana/cannabis products.
- Facial steam - fill a large bowl half full with boiling water & add ¼ cup apple cider vinegar, fresh or dried rosemary leaves, peppermint leaves & few drops of peppermint essential oil. With a towel over head, bend over bowl; breathe for about 5 to 15 minutes.
- Essential oils & reflexology to help ease headaches - birch, eucalyptus, helichrysum, lavender, oregano, peppermint, rosemary or sandalwood. Choose your own blend and add few drops on pillow, eye pillow, in diffuser, facial steam, spray, bath salts, body oil or lotion. Put a few drops on tissue, cotton ball or rub in palms of hand and hold up to nose. Mix 3 to 10 drops in 1 to 3 tablespoons any carrier oil & massage temples, over sinuses, webbed area between thumb and index finger, wrist pulse points, neck, shoulders and big toes.

Bath - add one of following to bath water; soak in warm to hot bath for about 15 to 45 minutes; suggestion to shower after to rinse off toxins:
- ½ cup to 1 cup apple cider vinegar, bentonite clay, sea salt or sole water or any combination.
- Bath bag - mix together crushed cinnamon sticks, slice ginger root, sea salt, eucalyptus leaves, rosemary leaves, lavender flowers, chamomile flowers or any combination. Put mixed blend into large press n' brew empty tea bags, muslin bags, old sock tied closed or large tea ball.
- ½ cup to 1 cup Bath Powder Blend or 1 to 4 tablespoons in foot bath (see DIY Recipes).

Internally
- Drink plenty of water - at least half your body weight in ounces daily; dehydration can cause headaches.
- Helps many people to balance hormones (see Hormone Imbalance).
- Possibly calcium and potassium deficiency (see Minerals & Vitamins).
- Feverfew & ginger gel.
- Bentonite clay water (see Bentonite Clay).

- Apple cider vinegar drink - 1 tablespoon each of apple cider vinegar and raw honey in glass of warm water; stir and drink 1 to 3 times a day.
- Menthol salve and/or lobelia oil - rub on temples, forehead and back of neck onto top of shoulders.
- Activated charcoal products.
- Rosemary and/or green tea with slice of ginger root and fresh mint leaves.
- Peppermint tea or peppermint essential oil pill supplement.
- Thai kratom powder - stir ½ teaspoon in glass of water or tea.
- Arnica products.

Herbs for Headaches
Butterbur, feverfew, ginger, kava kava, rosemary, sage, Thai kratom, vervain, white willow bark and wood betony

My Favorite Herbal Headache Combination
Butterbur, feverfew & Thai kratom.

Take herbs in powder, tincture, capsule or tea form - use all or any combination.

Heavy Metal Detox

Some heavy metal accumulation symptoms are black spots on gums or nails, brain issues, constipation, depression, digestive issues, easily frightened, fatigue, feeling weak & exhausted, gum & teeth issues, headaches, hormone imbalance, insomnia, low body temperature, metal taste in mouth, night sweats, mineral & vitamin deficiency, muscle & joint pain, teeth sensitivity, unexplained pain, tingly hands & feet.

Natural Suggestions to Help Prevent & Reduce Heavy Metal Accumulation in the Body
- Have mercury fillings removed from teeth safely.
- Saunas and hot yoga help sweat out toxins.
- Air purification systems.
- Dry skin brushing.
- Colon hydrotherapy.
- Ionic foot baths.
- Enemas - add ¼ cup of fresh cilantro juice or tea added to 2 quarts organic coffee enema.
- Massage therapy to promote circulation to help push out toxins.
- Chelation therapy is a treatment to bind and remove heavy metals and toxins from the blood.

- Switch to natural household and personal care products or make your own DIY products.
- Essential oils & reflexology to assist in removing heavy metals - mix 3 to 10 drops of cilantro essential oil in 1 to 3 tablespoons any carrier oil & massage into ankles, feet and wrists. Mix a few drops of clove essential oil in 1 tablespoon of any carrier oil into bottom of both feet before going to bed.

Bath - add one of the following to bath water; soak in warm to hot bath for about 15 to 45 minutes; suggestion to shower after to rinse off toxins:
- ½ cup to 2 cups bentonite clay, food grade diatomaceous earth, apple cider vinegar or any combination.
- ½ to 2 cups Bath Powder Blend (see DIY Recipes).
- Foot baths - 2 tablespoons to ½ cup of any suggestion above.

Internally
- Eat healthier, drink plenty of water and drink a whole food blender drink daily - consider including some of the foods listed below.
- Sulfur-rich foods - broccoli, Brussel sprout, cabbage, cauliflower, garlic and onion.
- Apple cider vinegar drink - 1 tablespoon each of apple cider vinegar and raw honey in glass of warm water; stir and drink 1 to 3 times a day.
- Bentonite clay, Pascalite clay or food grade diatomaceous earth - stir 1 teaspoon to 1 tablespoon in water, juice, coconut water, aloe vera juice and drink 1 to 3 times a day or mix in applesauce, yogurt or pudding
- Bentonite clay water (see Bentonite Clay).
- Grapefruit seed extract products - liquid made from the seeds, pulp and pith of grapefruit. It is used as a preservative and potent antioxidant while possessing antifungal, antibacterial and antiviral properties. It's been known to help with fungal or yeast infections, parasites, candida, diarrhea, nail fungus and strengthen immune system.
- Liquid chlorophyll.
- Activated charcoal products.
- MSM products.
- Omega fatty acids.
- Sea vegetables such as alaria, arame, bladderwrack, nori, dulse, ecklonia cava, Irish moss, kelp, kombu and wakame (can eat, powder form or supplement products).
- Spirulina & chlorella powder are blue/green algae containing high amounts of proteins, minerals, vitamins and mild chelators that bind to heavy metals to detoxify and remove them. Take in pill supplement,

tincture or add them to your powdered greens or whole food blender drink.
- Coral calcium supplements.
- Detox vegetable tea - produce suggestions include burdock leaf, cabbage leaf, cilantro leaf, collard green, dandelion green, fennel leaf, garlic clove, ginger root, horseradish root, kale leaf, leek, mustard green, onion, parsley leaf & turnip green. Simmer in gallon of water as many ingredients that you have available for about 30 minutes. Strain and drink cup of warm or cold tea 2 to 4 times a day. Keep in refrigerator for up to 1 week.
- Tamarind tea detox - bring 6 cups of water with 5 to 10 cut in half tamarind pods to a boil and simmer for 30 minutes. Remove pods and drink ½ cup of hot, room temperature or cold tea 2 to 4 times a day. Keep in refrigerator for up to 1 week.
- Super Tonic (see DIY Recipes).
- Watermelon Cleanse, *Essiac Tea* or *Master Cleanse* (see Colon/Cleanses).
- *Zeolite* supplement.

Herbal Help
- Powdered greens (see Powdered Greens).
- Eat fresh herbs, make tea or add to whole food blender drink. Herb suggestions include cilantro, clove, mint, parsley and oregano.

Take 2 to 4 times a day:
- Cilantro or coriander seed pills, tincture, tea or pesto.
- Drink green tea.
- Garlic - swallow 1 chopped garlic clove like a pill, or as a tincture, tea or pill supplement.
- Burdock root - as a tea or add slice of root in whole food blender drink or in pill supplement.
- Milk thistle in capsules - silymarin flavonoids in the milk thistle seeds stimulates liver cell production, to help flush out toxins and heavy metals.
- Milk thistle apple cider vinegar tincture; buy or make.

My Favorite Heavy Metal Removal Combination
Chlorella, cilantro, dandelion, spirulina & turmeric

Take herbs in powdered, tincture, capsule or tea form - use any combination.

These are Common Metals to Avoid
- Aluminum, which is found in aluminum foil, non-stick pots, pans, utensils, antiperspirants, antacids, aspirin, dentures, food preservatives, processed cheese, toothpastes and vaccines.
- Fluoride or sodium fluoride was patented in 1896 as an insecticide and is found in toothpastes, cleaning products, insecticides, rat poison and public drinking water supplies.
- Lead is found in canned foods, some makeups, paint, gasoline, batteries, pipes, ammunition, dishes and cosmetics.
- Mercury is found in dental fillings, thermometers, vaccines, light switches, some light bulbs, fish, shellfish and some high fructose corn syrups.

Hemorrhoids

Some causes are constipation, straining while eliminating stool & excessive sitting.
- Buy witch hazel cleansing cloths.
- Insert raw potato cut the size of small finger as a suppository.
- Enemas or colon hydrotherapy.
- Make Hemorrhoid Suppositories (see DIY Recipes).

Bath - add one of the following to bath water; soak in warm to hot bath or sitz bath for about 15 to 45 minutes 1 to 3 times a day:
- ½ to 1 cup bentonite clay, sea salt, witch hazel, Epsom salt or apple cider vinegar or any combination.
- ½ to 2 cups Bath Powder Blend (see DIY Recipes).

Apply to area a few times a day:
- Ice pack
- Aloe vera gel scraped from leaf.
- Goldenseal & myrrh salve.
- Vitamin E oil mixed with lavender and tea tree essential oils.
- Apple cider vinegar moistened cotton ball.
- Inside of banana peel.
- Cold cabbage leaves.
- Raw honey.
- Round gauze pads soaked in witch hazel or Hazel Toner and store in round jar few times a day (see DIY Recipes).
- Healing Salve (see DIY Recipes).
- Sanitizing Oil (see DIY Recipes).
- *Aloe Life Skin Gel.*

Internally
- Drink plenty of water to help prevent dried stools.
- Whole food blender drinks containing carrot, celery, ginger, kefir, parsley, prune and spinach.
- Probiotics such as probiotic supplements such as acidophilus, or *Good Belly* drink or *Innergy Biotic* drink.
- Eat 1 tablespoon of raw honey or add to herbal tea 3 times a day
- Herbal powder combination - bayberry, butchers broom, cayenne, white oak bark and witch hazel leaf. Encapsulate and take 2 to 4 capsules or take tincture, 3 squirts twice a day.

Itching

Apply a few times a day with fingertip, gauze pad or q-tip:
- Apple cider vinegar.
- Few drops of lavender essential oil mixed with 1 tablespoon of macadamia nut oil or carrier oil of your choice.
- Aloe vera gel scraped from leaf or *Aloe Life Skin Gel*.
- Witch hazel.
- Hazel Toner (see DIY Recipes).
- Sanitizing Oil (see DIY Recipes).
- Vitamin E oil.
- Chaparral oil, salve or tea.
- Fresh bruised plantain leaves.
- Piece of inside of banana peel.
- Manuka honey.
- Jewelweed salve, oil or tea ice cubes.
- Oatmeal - make normally; when oatmeal is warm, apply to affected area; after hardens, rinse or shower off.
- Buy or make itch oil or salve - chickweed & comfrey (see Herbal/Oil/Salves).
- Healing Salve (see DIY Recipes).
- Some natural itch cream or salve products online are *Terrasil* or *Dr. Christopher's Itch Ointment*.

Bath - add one of following to bath water; soak in warm to hot bath for about 15 to 45 minutes: suggestion to shower after to rinse off toxins:
- 1 to 2 cups oatmeal in large press n' brew empty tea bags, muslin bags, old sock tied closed or large tea ball.
- Bath bag - mix together chickweed leaves, comfrey leaves, plantain leaves, basil leaves, oatmeal, baking soda, bentonite clay or any

combination. Put mixed blend into large press n' brew empty tea bags, muslin bags, old sock tied closed or large tea ball.
- 1 to 2 cups apple cider vinegar or whole milk.
- ½ cup to 2 cups Bath Powder Blend (see DIY Recipes).

Compress - moisten cloth with herbal tea and apply for about 20 to 40 minutes:
- Herb suggestions include chaparral, chickweed, comfrey, echinacea, lobelia, myrrh and plantain.

Poultice - put fresh or dried herbs in muslin bag or press m' brew tea bags, moisten and apply for about 20 to 40 minutes:
- Herb suggestions include chaparral, chickweed, comfrey, echinacea, lobelia, myrrh and plantain.

Lice
- Apply oil generously to scalp and rub in. Use sesame, coconut, extra virgin olive oil, chaparral oil, neem oil or calendula oil.
- Cover with towel or shower cap. Leave on overnight.
- In the morning, wash hair and rinse with white vinegar or apple cider vinegar. Then, rinse with plain water and use nit comb.
- Repeat next night if needed. To help eliminate leftover unhatched eggs, reapplication after one week is recommended.

Lungs
- If you smoke cigarettes, then you should stop!
- Deep breathing - breath in slowly through nose for about 5 to 7 seconds; your stomach should expand. Hold breath for about 5 to 7 seconds or longer; then, slowly breathe all of the air out of mouth for about 5 to 10 seconds. Keep repeating. Do this anytime for about 5 to 10 minutes. Deep breathing is relaxing and good for stress, anxiety, adrenals and lungs.
- Himalayan sea salt inhaler.
- Menthol Salve on chest and upper back (see DIY Recipes).
- Cardiovascular exercises help cleanse lungs including biking, dancing, running, swimming and walking.
- Facial steam - fill a large bowl half full with boiling water & add aloe vera leaf, slice of ginger root, slice of horseradish root, sliced onions, osha root, fresh or dried mullein leaves, eucalyptus leaves & peppermint leaves. Use all ingredients or whatever you have available. With a towel over head, bend over bowl; breathe for about 5 to 15 minutes.

- Essential oils & reflexology to benefit the lungs - cedarwood, eucalyptus, frankincense, ginger, hyssop, marjoram, mullein, peppermint, pine, rose, ravensara, rosemary, rosewood, sandalwood, spruce, tea tree or thyme. Choose your own blend and use in diffuser, spray or add to above facial steam. Put a few drops on tissue, cotton ball or rub in palms of hand and hold up to nose. Add 3 to 10 drops in 1 to 3 tablespoons any carrier oil & massage into chest, upper back, belly and both feet.

Internally
- Omega fatty acids.
- Combine 1 tablespoon apple cider vinegar and 1 teaspoon baking soda in glass of juice, water or herbal tea and drink 2 to 3 times a day.
- Cook bunch of asparagus in 1 gallon of boiling water for about 15 minutes, remove asparagus and drink 1 cup of asparagus water 2 to 3 times a day.
- Squeeze juice of whole lemon or lime with a 1 tablespoon of raw honey in glass of warm water and drink 2 to 3 times a day.
- Take 1 tablespoon of raw honey after each meal or chew on honeycomb.
- Onions are an expectorant - soak sliced onions and garlic in raw honey overnight; take 1 tablespoon of infused honey a few times a day.
- Mushroom supplement products or tea.
- Super Tonic (see DIY Recipes.)

Herbal Help
- Lobelia alcohol tincture - help lungs release mucus.
- Fresh grated ginger root tea - 1 tablespoon grated ginger into cup of hot water, let steep for about 10 minutes; optional to add lemon juice, raw honey, cinnamon stick, garlic clove, pinch of cayenne or whole clove.
- Mullein and peppermint tea.
- Osha root - chew on piece of osha root, osha tincture, tea or use osha spray.

Herbs to Benefit Lungs
Astragalus, brigham tea, chaparral, coltsfoot, echinacea, elecampane, eucalyptus, fenugreek, gentian, ginger, goldenseal, horehound, hyssop, licorice root, lobelia, lungwort, marshmallow root, mullein, myrrh, oregano, osha, peppermint, plantain, pleurisy root, red root, rosemary, sea buckthorn, spikenard, thyme, yarrow and wild cherry

My Favorite Herbal Lung Combination
Echinacea, lobelia, mullein, pleurisy root & marshmallow root.

Take herbs in powder, tincture, capsule or tea form - use any combination.

Lymphatic System

Made up of glands, lymph nodes, thymus gland, spleen & tonsils. Carries the toxins away from tissues & cells to the blood to be filtered out by the liver & kidneys to strengthen immune system.

- Deep breathing - breath in slowly through nose for about 5 to 7 seconds; your stomach should expand. Hold breath for about 5 to 7 seconds or longer; then, slowly breathe all of the air out of mouth for about 5 to 10 seconds. Keep repeating. Do this anytime for about 5 to 10 minutes. Deep breathing is relaxing and good for stress, anxiety, adrenals and lungs.
- Physical activity - jumping on a trampoline for 5 to 10 minutes daily benefits lymphatic system, also aerobic exercise, yoga, light hand weights, walking and stretching.
- Dry skin brushing.
- Inversion table or sauna.
- Foot reflexology or foot zoning.
- Acupuncture, lymph massage or any massage helps.
- Stay away from underwire bras; they can block the lymphatic flow. Also helps to wear loose clothing.
- Stand on your head for 2 to 10 minutes.
- Hot and cold showers - alternate 3 to 7 times and always end with cold, or switch from hot and cold tubs, or jacuzzi to cool pool for more circulation.
- Medical marijuana/cannabis products.
- Menthol Salve (see DIY Recipes).
- Essential oils to benefit lymphatic system are geranium, grapefruit, lemon, orange, sandalwood and tangerine. Mix 3 to 6 drops essential oils of your choice in 1 tablespoon carrier oil of your choice and rub into neck, chest, under arms and between breasts to stimulate lymphatic drainage.

Internally
- Eat healthier & drink plenty of water.
- Drink lemon water first thing in morning on an empty stomach daily.
- Apple cider vinegar drink - 1 tablespoon each of apple cider vinegar and raw honey in glass of warm water; stir and drink 1 to 3 times a day.
- Super Tonic (see DIY Recipes).
- Infection Fighter Herbal Tincture (see DIY Recipes).
- Watermelon Cleanse, *Essiac Tea* or *Master Cleanse* (see Colon/Cleanses).

Herbal Help

- Powdered greens (see Powdered Greens).
- Herbal tea - herbal suggestions include astragalus, blue violet, bupleurum, cleavers, devil's claw, echinacea, goldenseal, manjistha, moringa, nettle, red clover blossoms and wild indigo root.
- Spirulina and/or chlorella products.

Nausea

- Reflexology - measure three fingers up on inside of forearm from bend of wrist, and then apply pressure with thumb for about 1 minute.
- Inhale peppermint essential oil by putting a few drops on tissue, cotton ball or rub in palms of hand and hold up to nose.
- Acupuncture or meditation.

Internally

- Cut open lemon and inhale or bite into lemon.
- Peppermint gum or candy.
- Drink lemon water first thing in morning on empty stomach.
- Medical marijuana/cannabis products.
- Raw potato juice - grate potato and squeeze through cloth; drink 1 to 2 tablespoons of potato juice in 1 cup of warm water.
- Activated charcoal products.
- Apple cider vinegar drink - 1 tablespoon each of apple cider vinegar and raw honey in glass of warm water; stir and drink 1 to 3 times a day.
- CBD products.
- 1 to 3 drops of therapeutic ginger or peppermint essential oil in glass of water or herbal tea.
- Ginger, lemon and/or peppermint essential oils mixed in any carrier oil; then rub on abdomen clockwise, both feet, wrists, temples and behind ears.

Herbal Help

- Fresh grated ginger root tea - 1 tablespoon grated ginger into cup of hot water, let steep for about 10 minutes; optional to add lemon juice, raw honey, cinnamon stick, garlic clove, pinch of cayenne or whole clove
- Ginger pill supplement, chew on ginger root or crystallized ginger chews.
- Motion sickness - 2 ginger pill supplement before traveling and again 2 hours later.
- Cinnamon water - 1 teaspoon cinnamon powder in room temperature glass of water.

- Hot cinnamon tea - 1 teaspoon cinnamon powder, few whole cloves and cinnamon stick in cup of hot water.
- Chew fresh peppermint leaves.
- Drink chamomile or peppermint tea throughout day.

Herbs to Help with Nausea
Catnip, chamomile, cinnamon, dandelion, fennel, wild lettuce, ginger, licorice root, peppermint, nutmeg and red raspberry

Take herbs in powder, tincture, capsule or tea form - use any combination.

Sleep

Important to get 6 to 9 hours of sleep a night. Sleeping is one way our body heals, repairs & strengthens the immune system. The following suggestions are known to help reduce stress, anxiety, calm nerves & promote good sleep.

- Good to go to bed around same time each night.
- Avoid taking long naps although 20 to 30 minutes can improve memory, alertness and performance.
- For most people, the room should be dark, cool and quiet at bedtime.
- Maintain a healthy body weight & stay hydrated.
- Avoid a heavy meal before bed. Your body starts to warm up to start digesting the meal. Your body should be cooling down to go to sleep.
- Avoid fluorescent lighting which can throw our body's time clock off.
- Exposure to sunlight in the morning will activate the pineal gland to boost serotonin & melatonin levels to help you sleep better.
- Feng shui helps create a harmonious balance of energies in any given space. It promotes health, prosperity and good fortune for anyone using that space. Position the bed away from corners of bedroom, it should be easily accessible from both sides. Windows should be at side of the bed. Avoid water features, electrical and exercise equipment in bedroom. Remove clutter in bedroom and open window during day to get fresh air.
- Sound therapy to promote relaxation - listen to calming music, white noise, pink noise, electroencephalogram music, tuning forks or singing bowls.
- EFT or Emotion Freedom Technique - a process of tapping areas of the body to clear out negative energy blockages. Helps with pain, stress, fear, inflammation, depression, anxiety and headaches. EFT is easy to learn and easy to do on yourself.
- Meditation for about 20 minutes a day to help quiet the mind.
- Sage smudging.
- Acupuncture, chiropractic or reiki.

- Massage therapy to help loosen muscles, increase circulation and relieve tension and stress.
- Reflexology, shiatsu or Indian head massage.
- Yoga, stretching, tai chi, qigong or massage feet a few hours before bed.
- Scalp wire massager.
- Biofeedback mat.
- Floatation tank therapy.
- CBD products.
- Deep breathing - breath in slowly through nose for about 5 to 7 seconds; your stomach should expand. Hold breath for about 5 to 7 seconds or longer; then, slowly breathe all of the air out of mouth for about 5 to 10 seconds. Keep repeating. Do this anytime for about 5 to 10 minutes. Deep breathing is relaxing and good for stress, anxiety, adrenals and lungs.
- Herbal relaxing eye pillow - use half chamomile & lavender flowers with flaxseeds; buy or make.
- Lavender bags - fill muslin bags, large press n' brew empty tea bags or tied off sock with whole dried lavender flowers. Place under your pillow, use as bath bag, in dryer to soften and freshen clothes or as drawer sachet.
- Cut yellow onion and keep in glass jar. Before sleep or when you wake up at night, open jar and inhale.
- Himalayan salt lamps produce negative ions or invisible molecules which we inhale similar to those nature produces like being in the mountains, near waterfalls or the beach and works as a natural ionizer to cleanse the air. They produce positive biochemical reactions that increase serotonin levels to help alleviate depression and stress. Salt lamps are known to improve sleep, help give a sense of well-being, decrease allergy symptoms, neutralize the effects of electrical devices and cleanse negative energy.
- Put a stone or crystal under pillow or on floor under bed, one at each corner and one in the middle of the bed. Stone suggestions are amethyst, hematite, jade, malachite or smoky quartz.
- Essential oils & reflexology for relaxing, anxiety and stress - bergamot, chamomile, clary sage, geranium, jasmine, lavender, lemon balm, neroli, patchouli, rose or sandalwood. Choose your own blend and add drops on pillow, eye pillow, in diffuser, spray, bath salts, body oil or lotion. Put a few drops on tissue, cotton ball or rub in palms of hand and hold up to nose. Mix 3 to 10 drops of essential oils of your choice in 1 to 3 tablespoons any carrier oil & massage arch of feet, wrists, neck and temples.
- Listening to *Sleep With Me Podcast* on your phone - he tells boring bedtime stories.

Bath - add one of following to bath water; soak in warm to hot bath for about 15 to 45 minutes. Any warm to hot bath can promote sleep as the cooling down process will promote deeper sleep:
- Aromatherapy baths salts or oil - mix 10 to 20 drops lavender essential oil or above essential oils of choice in ¼ to 1 cup of any carrier oil, honey or sea salt (see Essential Oils).
- Bath bag - mix together ¼ cup each of lavender flowers, chamomile flowers, rosebuds, rose petals, sea salt, bentonite clay or any combination. Put mixed blend into large press n' brew empty tea bags, muslin bags, old sock tied closed or large tea ball.
- ½ cup to 1 cup magnesium powder, sea salt, sole water.
- ½ cup to 2 cups Bath Powder Blend (see DIY Recipes).
- 1 to 2 cups of *Dr. Teal's Epsom Salts.*

Internally
- Coral calcium contains minerals that might be lacking to help you sleep. Also helps with nightmares and bedwetting.
- Melatonin - a hormone secreted at night by the pineal gland that helps regulates sleep patterns.
  The production goes up at night to make you sleepy and drops in the morning to wake you up. Taking melatonin pill supplement may reset your body clock when you working graveyard shift. For jet lag, take recommended dose when it gets dark starting the day before traveling; continue on the day of travel and three days after, especially when traveling west coast to east coast.
- Tryptophan - an amino acid important for brain function which can help improve quality of sleep, helps blood circulation, hormones and helps the body produce serotonin and melatonin. Food sources like beans, cheese, eggs, lentils, nuts, oats, pineapple, salmon, seeds and turkey.
- L-theanine or GABA - amino acids that help reduce anxiety, mental and physical stress.
- Eat natural sugar about 4 hours before bed - some suggestions are banana, kiwi or watermelon.
- Possible magnesium deficiency (see Minerals & Vitamins).
- Medical marijuana/cannabis products.
- Eat a banana or boil a whole banana for 10 minutes with the peel on to make a tea. Drink the tea and then eat the whole boiled banana; slice it up peel and all; then sprinkle on some cinnamon and/or raw honey.
- Helps many people to balance hormones (see Hormone Imbalance).

- *Natural Calm* is a powdered magnesium supplement known to help relax muscles, promote sleep and helps prevent muscle twitching, leg cramps and constipation.
- Flower essence - *Bach Rescue Night* & *Rescue Remedy* products.

Drink about 1 hour before bedtime:
- ½ cup of kefir with tablespoon of raw honey.
- 8 ounces of sugar free cherry juice.
- 1 ounce of black cherry concentrate in glass of water.
- 1 cup of warm water with 1 tablespoon of raw honey after evening meal.
- Chamomile tea or tincture. Helps to relieve nightmares, improves sleep, digestion and rebuilds nerve endings.
- Nutmeg or clove powder - 1 teaspoon in cup of warm whole milk or kefir.
- *Essiac Tea* - drinking about ½ to 1 cup of decoction at night.

Herbs to Help Relax and Calm Anxiety, Stress and Nerves
Ashwagandha, basil, blue vervain, California poppy, catnip, chamomile, damiana, ecklonia cava, gotu kola, holy basil, hops, jasmine, kava kava, lavender, lemon balm, licorice root, linden flower, magnolia bark, mugwort, muira puama, nutmeg, passionflower, rhodiola, schizandra, skullcap, St. John's Wort, Thai kratom, valerian root, vervain, wild lettuce and wood betony

My Favorite Herbal Sleep Combination
Chamomile, kava kava, valerian root & wild lettuce.

My Favorite Herbal Anxiety and/or Stress Combination
Kava kava, hops, holy basil, licorice root & St. John's Wort.

Take herbs in powder, tincture, capsule or tea form - use any combination.

Dried Herbal Relaxing Tea Combination
- California Poppy Flower
- Catnip Leaf
- Chamomile Flower
- Jasmine Flower
- Lavender Flower
- Passion Flower
- Valerian Root
- Wild Lettuce Leaf

Use all above ingredients or any above dried herbal combination. Mix ingredients together and store in closed container. 1 tablespoon dried herbal combination in small press n' brew empty tea bags, tea ball or mesh strainer per cup of boiling water. Steep for 15 to 30 minutes and drink 1 to 3 cups a day.

Sore Throat

- Menthol Salve on neck and chest (see DIY Recipes).
- Throat Gargle (see DIY Recipes)
- Moisten cloth or paper towel with warm sole water and wrap cloth around neck for half hour 2 to 3 times a day.
- Onion and carrots poultice - place a few sliced or chopped onions and carrots into tube sock tied closed; moisten with apple cider vinegar, wrap around neck for up to 1 hour.
- Facial steam - fill a large bowl half full with boiling water & add ¼ cup apple cider vinegar, fresh or dried peppermint leaves, eucalyptus leaves, slice of ginger root, jalapeno pepper, aloe vera leaf, sliced garlic cloves, few whole cloves, few drops each of ravansara & thyme essential oils. Use all ingredients or whatever you have available. With a towel over head, bend over bowl; breathe for about 5 to 15 minutes.
- Oil pulling draws out toxins and bacteria by swishing 1 tablespoon of sesame seed oil or coconut oil back and forth, front and back through teeth for 5 to 20 minutes; spit out and rinse.
- Mix together 1 tablespoon of cinnamon and 1 tablespoon of coconut oil; rub on chest and neck.
- Essential oils & reflexology to fight infections - black pepper, cinnamon, eucalyptus, garlic, ginger, lemon, oregano, peppermint, ravansara, sage, rosemary, tea tree or thyme. Mix 3 to 10 drops of essential oils of your choice in 1 to 3 tablespoons any carrier oil & massage neck, chest, behind ears, toes and joint area of toes.

Internally

- Infection Fighter Herbal Tincture - take 3 squirts every 1 to 3 hours or squirt into warm herbal tea (see DIY Recipe).
- Hot honey - 1 tablespoon raw honey with ¼ teaspoon of cayenne or ginger powder; take straight or add to hot water or herbal tea.
- Honey gel tea - fill jar with 3 parts sliced lemons, 1 part sliced ginger root and then fill jar with raw honey; and place in the refrigerator. The ingredients will turn into a gel. Make tea with 1 tablespoon of gel and cup of hot water. Can last 3 months in the refrigerator.
- Combo tea - combine 1 tablespoon raw honey, ¼ to ½ teaspoon cinnamon powder, juice of half lemon, 2 slices of ginger root and dash of cayenne powder in a cup of hot water or green tea; drink 2 to 3 times a day.
- Hot throat syrup - mix ¼ cup of raw honey, ¼ cup apple cider vinegar, ¼ teaspoon each of cayenne and clove powder; take 1 tablespoon as needed.

- Herbal tea - herb suggestions include bugleweed, echinacea, ginger, goldenseal, licorice, mullein and red root. Use one or any combination..
- Mix 1 ounce of aloe vera juice or gel with 1 teaspoon of mucilage herbs like slippery elm bark powder, coltsfoot or marshmallow root powder; drink to soothe and coat esophagus to enhance healing.
- Chew on slice of licorice root.
- Chew on piece of osha root, osha tincture, tea or use osha spray.
- *Fisherman's Friend* lozenges or *Throat Coat* tea.

Gargle 1 teaspoon to 1 tablespoon for about 30 seconds to a minute and spit out every couple of hours until feeling better:

- Apple cider vinegar - 3 tablespoons apple cider vinegar in 4 ounces of water or herbal tea.
- Super Tonic (see DIY Recipes).
- Throat Gargle (see DIY Recipes).
- Himalayan sea salt or sole water - 2 tablespoons in ¼ cup of warm water.
- Colloidal silver.
- Fresh sage tea gargle - 1 cup of boiling water over sage; steep 10 minutes.
- Add 2 to 5 drops of above therapeutic essential oils of your choice to ¼ cup of warm water.

Toenail Fungus or Athlete's Foot

Foot bath suggestions - soak feet in warm to hot foot bath for about 15 to 30 minutes; soak feet daily till gone:

- Herbal foot bath tea - herb suggestions include chaparral, garlic, echinacea, myrrh, oregano, pau d'arco, thyme or any combination. Put 2 tablespoons of herb blend in press n' brew empty tea bags, muslin bags, old sock tied closed or small tea ball. Optional to add a few drops of below mentioned essential oils.
- ¼ to 1 cup apple cider vinegar or hydrogen peroxide.
- 2 tablespoons each of diatomaceous earth powder & apple cider vinegar.
- ¼ cup to ½ cup Bath Powder Blend (see DIY Recipes).

Apply a few times a day with fingertip, gauze pad or q-tip:

- Chaparral oil, salve or tea.
- Healing Salve (see DIY Recipes).
- Sanitizing Oil (see DIY Recipes).
- Rub clove of garlic, oil or tincture on feet.
- Grapefruit seed extract products.
- Emu oil.
- Apple cider vinegar or hydrogen peroxide.

- Essential oils to attack toenail fungus by applying 1 to 3 drops of undiluted cinnamon, clove, garlic, lemon, oregano or tea tree essential oil on toenail or add 3 to 10 drops essential oils of your choice in 1 tablespoon of carrier oil of your choice and massage feet, toenails and between toes.

Sprinkle 1 to 2 tablespoons of bentonite clay or food grade diatomaceous earth in socks before going to bed or anytime.

Toothache or Gum Pain

- Salt gargle - mix 1 teaspoon sea salt in ¼ cup warm water and gargle about 1 tablespoons for 1 minute 3 to 5 times a day. Optional to add 3 drops of therapeutic grade clove essential oil.
- Mouthwash (see DIY Recipes).
- Swish 1 tablespoon of food grade hydrogen peroxide or 3% hydrogen peroxide in mouth for 1 minute few times a day; spit out and rinse.
- Add a few drops of clove, helichrysum, myrrh or oregano therapeutic grade essential oils to mouthwash or tooth powder.
- Swish cooled peppermint tea in mouth for 1 minute 3 to 5 times a day; then spit out.
- Oil pulling draws out toxins and bacteria by swishing 1 tablespoon of sesame seed oil or coconut oil back and forth, front and back through teeth for 5 to 20 minutes; spit out and rinse.
- Wet black tea bag on area.
- Abscessed tooth - mix 1 teaspoon each of bentonite clay, activated charcoal powder, slippery elm bark, colloidal silver and 2 drops each of clove and oregano essential oil. Wrap up about ½ teaspoon at a time in small piece of cloth and or press n' brew empty tea bags. Leave on sore tooth and gums up to an hour and then throw away. Apply 3 to 5 times a day. Will help pull infection out and help with pain.
- Gum infection - myrrh, goldenseal, turmeric and/or white oak bark herbal tea gargle or place tea bag on gums.
- Reflexology - apply pressure into joint area between thumb and forefinger where they meet on both hands and hold for 1 to 3 minutes.
- Gentle tooth gel - brush with *Miracle II* neutralizer gel.

Apply a few times a day with fingertip, gauze pad or q-tip:
- Slice of garlic clove.
- Rub on medical marijuana oil or butter.

- 1 to 2 drops of undiluted therapeutic grade essential oil and massage into gums where it hurts, such as clove, helichrysum, myrrh or oregano. Will numb and calm inflammation to help blood flow.
- Mix 3 drops of above therapeutic grade essential oil of choice with 1 tablespoon of extra virgin olive oil or aloe vera gel scraped from a leaf.
- Rub ice cube into webbed area between thumb and forefinger on both hands or ice pack on jaw over painful area.
- Herbal paste - ¼ teaspoon of turmeric and/or myrrh powder mixed with enough water to make a paste.

Wounds & Cuts

- First thing to do is to clean wound with soap and water.
- Fresh comfrey or plantain leaves - moisten leaves and apply to area (plantain leaves are known as nature's band aid and comfrey leaves are known as a bone healer).
- Apply herbal tea bag or compress to area using fresh, dried or powdered herbs. Herb suggestions include chamomile, calendula, chaparral, comfrey, lavender, lemon balm, myrrh, oregano, parsley, plantain, pau d'arco and thyme.

Buy or make a spray using:
- 1 part apple cider vinegar & 3 parts distilled water.
- Colloidal silver.
- Sanitizing Spray (see Essential Oils/Favorite Uses).

Apply a few times a day with fingertip, gauze pad or q-tip:
- Apple cider vinegar.
- Raw honey or mix honey with myrrh, yarrow, oregano or cayenne powder.
- Aloe vera gel scrap from leaf or *Aloe Life Skin Gel.*
- Colloidal silver liquid, cream, salve or gel.
- Calendula oil, cream, salve, ointment.
- Medical marijuana/cannabis products.
- Chaparral and/or oil, salve or tea.
- Garlic oil, salve or tea.
- Lavender and/or lobelia herbal oil.
- Black salve (great for fungal infections).
- Vitamin E oil (great for scars)
- Tea tree or neem essential oil.
- Sole Water (see Himalayan Sea Salt).
- Hazel Toner (see DIY Recipes).
- Sanitizing Oil (see DIY Recipes).

- Healing Salve (see DIY Recipes).
- Essential oils to enhance wound healing by mixing 3 to 10 drops of essential oils like davana, lemon, oregano or tea tree in 1 tablespoon any carrier oil.

Yeast/Fungal Infection
Candida & Parasites.

Some yeast overgrowth symptoms are allergies, athlete's foot, bloated abdomen, blurred vision, brain fog, constipation, chronic fatigue, dandruff, depression, diarrhea, drippy nose, drooling while sleeping, dry mouth, ear & sinus infections, ear noise or ringing in ears, eczema, eye floaters, fibromyalgia, gas, grind teeth, heartburn, high blood sugar levels, high cholesterol levels, insomnia, itchy ears, joint & soft tissue inflammation, low body temperature, muscle weakness, oral thrush, poor digestion, rectal itching, recurring vaginal yeast or bacterial infections, skin rashes, toenail fungus, sugar & carb cravings.

Natural Suggestions to Help Against Yeast & Parasites
- Tongue cleaning - when you are sleeping, your body is busy clearing out toxins. Some toxins are found as white, yellow, green or brown coating on tongue. Clean tongue using a tongue scraper first thing in the morning.
- Dry skin brushing.
- Ionic foot baths.
- Enemas or colon hydrotherapy.
- For skin issues (see Wounds & Cuts).
- *Para Zapper.*

Bath - add one of following to bath water; soak in very warm to hot bath for about 15 to 45 minutes; suggestion to shower after to rinse off toxins:
- ½ cup to 2 cups apple cider vinegar & ½ cup food grade diatomaceous earth or bentonite clay.
- ½ to 2 cups Bath Powder Blend (see DIY Recipes).

Internally
- Eat healthier & drink plenty of water.
- Whole food blender drink daily - ingredient suggestions are almond, kefir, dragon fruit, ginger, kale, lemon, onion, papaya seed, pineapple & stem, papaya, pomegranate seed, pumpkin seed, spinach and whole clove.
- Garlic - swallow 1 to 3 chopped cloves like a pill or as a tincture, tea or pill supplement.

- Grapefruit seed extract products.
- Bentonite clay or food grade diatomaceous earth powder - stir 1 teaspoon to 1 tablespoon in water, juice, coconut water or aloe vera juice. Drink 1 to 3 times a day about a half hour before meals or mix in applesauce or yogurt.
- Colloidal silver.
- Oregano essential oil pill supplement.
- Copper infused water - store water for 8 hours to overnight in 100% copper vessel, for instance a pitcher, mug or water bottle and drink 1 to 2 glasses a day for its anti-inflammatory, antibacterial and antiviral properties.
- Enemas - using organic coffee, garlic, pau d'arco or chaparral tea
- Chia seed drink - 2 tablespoons chia seeds in pint jar filled with distilled water and juice of 1 or 2 lemons. Drink all at once or throughout day.
- Apple cider vinegar - 1 tablespoon 2 to 3 times a day in a glass of water.
- Kombucha mushroom tea; buy or make.
- Chaparral, wormwood and/or pau d'arco tea cleanse - use dried herbs; fill pint jar ¼ full of herb(s), fill with hot water, let sit for 1 to 8 hours and drink 1 pint a day for 2 weeks.
- Detox vegetable tea - produce suggestions include burdock leaf, cabbage leaf, cilantro leaf, collard green, dandelion green, fennel leaf, garlic clove, ginger root, horseradish root, kale leaf, leek, mustard green, onion, parsley leaf & turnip green. Simmer in gallon of water as many ingredients that you have available for about 30 minutes. Strain, drink cup of warm or cold tea 2 to 3 times a day. Keep in refrigerator for up to 3 days.
- Cut skin off papaya, cut up fruit and ferment in 2 cups apple cider vinegar for 2 days; then drink 2 ounces twice a day till gone.
- Super Tonic (see DIY Recipes).
- Infection Fighter Herbal Tincture (see DIY Recipes).
- Watermelon Cleanse, *Essiac Tea* or *Master Cleanse* (see Colon/Cleanses).
- Probiotics such as probiotic supplements such as acidophilus, or *Good Belly* drink or *Innergy Biotic* drink.
- Some good herbal supplement products online are *TriGuard Plus, Candisol, Solaray - Yeast Cleanse* or *Kyolic - Candida Cleanse.*

Antifungal Detox Herbs

Black walnut hulls, cajeput, cassia, cayenne, cinnamon bark, chaparral, Chinese goldthread, clove, echinacea, fennel, garlic, ginger, goldenseal, horseradish, juniper berry, myrrh, neem, olive leaf, Oregon grape, pau d'arco, spikenard, sarsaparilla, thyme, white oak bark and yellow dock root

Parasite Detox Herbs

Black walnut hulls, cayenne, Chinese goldthread, clove, epazote, garlic, ginger, male fern, milkweed, pau d'arco, pumpkin seed, turmeric and wormwood

My Favorite Antifungal/Parasite Herbal Combination

Black walnut hulls, cayenne, chaparral, clove, olive leaf, pau d'arco & wormwood

Take herbs in powdered, tincture, capsule or tea form - use any combination.

DIY RECIPES FOR PERSONAL CARE & BATH PRODUCTS

These are ideas & suggestions. You can change or adjust as you need or desire.

Before you start any DIY recipe; you should clean and sanitize preparation tools. Sanitizing helps prevent contamination and allows the DIY product to last longer. Soak all preparation tools such as empty bottles, jars, bowls, droppers, funnels and utensils in a bowl with hydrogen peroxide or rubbing alcohol for a few minutes and let them dry completely. You can also put hydrogen peroxide or rubbing alcohol in a spray bottle and spray preparation tools, jars and containers and let them dry completely before using. Remember to label all containers with product name, and maybe the date made and list of ingredients.

Bath Powder Blend
Ingredients:
- 2 to 3 cups powdered Himalayan sea salt
- 2 to 3 cups bentonite clay
- ½ cup powdered ginger
- ½ cup powdered apple cider vinegar

How to Make & Use
- Mix ingredients together, break up any lumps with a fork and store in closed container.
- Add ½ cup to 2 cups in a very warm to hot bath water.
- 1 to 4 tablespoons in a foot bath.
- Soak for about 15 to 45 minutes.
- Helps to relax muscles and release toxins.
- Reduces inflammation and pain while absorbing the nutrients contained in the ingredients.
- Suggestion to shower after to rinse off toxins.

Cellulite or Circulation Scrub
Ingredients:
- ½ cup fine to coarse sea salt or raw coconut sugar
- ½ cup coffee grounds

- 1 teaspoon of powdered herb or herb combination. Herb suggestions include cinnamon, ginger and kelp
- ½ teaspoon cayenne powder
- 1 to 3 tablespoons of carrier oil of your choice such as almond, argan, coconut, emu, grapeseed, hemp, jojoba, olive, safflower or sesame

How to Make & Use
- Mix ingredients together in a bowl and store rest in closed container.
- Rub 1 to 3 tablespoons into each desired area like the legs, arms or belly, in a circular motion for about 10 to 15 minutes.
- Optional to do light dry skin brushing first.

Cough Syrups

Herbal cough syrup ingredients:
- 1 cup distilled water (use less water for a thicker syrup)
- 1 cup raw honey
- ¼ to ½ cup of herb combination. Herb suggestions include cherry bark, cinnamon sticks, horehound, thyme, elderberries, elecampane, licorice root, garlic, ginger, goldenseal, hyssop, mullein, osha root, peppermint, red root, sarsaparilla, spikenard, yerba santa and whole cloves; use fresh, dried or powdered herbs

Example herbal blend combination - elderberries, horehound and mullein.

How to Make & Use
- Make herbal tea with distilled water and herbs in crock-pot (can also use stainless steel pot or glass pot on stove).
- Use high setting on crock-pot for about 1 hour.
- Turn off crock-pot to cool down infusion to strain.
- Put strained infusion back into crock-pot.
- Add 1 cup raw honey; under age 2 can use blackstrap molasses or maple syrup.
- Optional to add ¼ teaspoon of cayenne powder or ¼ cup whiskey or brandy.
- Mix well while simmering a few minutes.
- Store in glass jar & keep in refrigerator or cool dry place for about 2 months.

Other simple raw honey cough syrups:
1. Mix ¼ cup raw honey ⅛ cup apple cider vinegar; can also add juice of ½ lemon and pinch of cayenne powder to taste.

2. Mix ¼ cup raw honey & 1 teaspoon cinnamon powder.
3. Make garlic honey by covering peeled garlic cloves with raw honey and leave overnight, remove garlic next day; or chop up and leave in honey.

Dosage for cough syrups:
- Children - 1 teaspoon every 3 to 6 hours
- Adults - 1 tablespoon every 3 to 6 hours

Deodorant

Ingredients:
- 1 to 2 tablespoons of coconut oil

1 tablespoon of each powder:
- Arrowroot
- Baking soda
- Bentonite clay
- Corn starch

Optional to add 2 to 3 drops of essential oils of like cinnamon, grapefruit, lemon, orange, oregano, sage, thyme or tea tree.

How to Make & Use
- Mix dry ingredients together in a jar; then add 1 to 2 tablespoons of coconut oil & essential oils to the consistency you prefer. The consistency of smooth apple sauce works well. Apply to underarms with fingers.

Garlic Oil - has antibiotic, antibacterial and antiviral properties.

Ingredients:
- 1 cup extra virgin olive oil.
- 2 to 3 whole garlic clove bulbs.

How to Make & Use
- Coarsely chop garlic cloves or blend garlic cloves in blender.
- Fill canning jar or glass jar with a lid about ⅓ full with blended garlic.
- Then fill jar with extra virgin olive oil.
- Cover and put jar on a windowsill in the sunlight if possible, otherwise just keep jar on counter or in cabinet.
- Shake jar daily for 3 days.
- Strain and store in refrigerator for about a month.
- Some uses include cooking, salad dressing and marinade.
- Medicinal purposes mentioned or suggested throughout book.

Hazel Toner

Ingredients:
- 1 cup witch hazel.
- ¼ cup dried calendula flowers.
- ¼ cup dried lavender flowers.
- 8 to 12 drops each of tea tree and lavender essential oil.

How to Make & Use
- Put flowers and witch hazel into canning jar or glass jar with a lid.
- Cover and keep jar on counter; steep for about 4 weeks, shake or stir daily.
- Strain and stir essential oils into infused witch hazel.
- Pour liquid into bottle with a lid, pump bottle or spray bottle.
- Some uses include facial toner, aftershave or as an antiseptic by moistening cotton ball or gauze pad to use on wounds, bites, rashes and hemorrhoids.
- Make Hazel Toner Pads by soaking round gauze pads with Hazel Toner, store pads in round jar to keep moist, to be ready to use when needed.
- Medicinal purposes mentioned or suggested throughout book.

Healing Herbal Salve

Ingredients:
- 1 cup extra virgin olive oil.
- 2 ounces beeswax (vegan alternative is carnauba wax).
- ¼ cup powdered herb combination. Herb suggestions include chaparral, comfrey, echinacea, lobelia, myrrh and plantain.

Optional to add a few drops of vitamin E oil and/or essential oils like clove, davana, lemon, oregano, thyme or tea tree.

How to Make & Use
- Extra virgin olive oil & herbs on warm or low setting in small crock-pot.
- Stir and steep for 1 to 7 days; stir a few times a day; the longer you steep, the stronger the oil.
- When oil is ready, strain oil through muslin cloth, muslin bag, cheesecloth or coffee filter by hand into bowl, or use a tincture press.
- Put strained herbal oil back or use previously prepared herbal oil into crock-pot and add beeswax. Once melted and blended, turn crock-pot off to cool off.
- If adding vitamin E oil and/or essential oils, do so now.

- Stir to blend in oils; pour warm liquid salve into jars to harden. If using plastic containers, be careful oil is not too hot or your containers could melt.
- Start by filling only one jar to harden to test the consistency of salve. If too hard, put back into crock-pot and add some extra virgin olive oil; if it is too loose, add some more wax.
- Some uses include bites, burns, rashes and wounds.
- Medicinal purposes mentioned or suggested throughout book.

Hemorrhoid Suppositories

Ingredients:

- ¼ cup coconut oil, cocoa butter, mango butter or kokum butter.
- ¼ cup herb combination. Herb suggestions include cayenne, comfrey, mullein, plantain, slippery elm bark, turmeric, yarrow, white oak bark and witch hazel; herbs in powder form is preferred.

Optional to add 2 to 5 drops of essential oils like chamomile, cypress, davana, frankincense, geranium, juniper, helichrysum, lavender, rosemary, tea tree or sandalwood.

How to Make & Use

- Mix herbs you have together in a bowl with enough butter or oils into a thick paste.
- Put paste into refrigerator to firm up.
- Roll firmed up paste into small cones like half the size of your small finger.
- Wrap each one in wax paper or parchment paper.
- Or layer cones on wax paper or parchment paper in a closed container.
- Put container in refrigerator or freezer to get hard before using one.
- Store rest in the freezer for future use.
- Suppository needs to be cold and inserted right away or will melt from heat of your hands; then leave in.

Infection Fighter Herbal Tincture

Ingredients:

- 4 ounces food grade vegetable glycerin.
- 4 ounces distilled water.
- 1 ounce powdered herb combination. Herb suggestions include astragalus, echinacea, elderberries, goldenseal, myrrh and yarrow.

How to Make & Use
- Put all ingredients into canning jar or glass jar with a lid, shake or stir to mix together.
- Cover, label and date. Keep jar on counter or in cabinet; let steep for about 2 weeks, shake or stir 1 to 2 times a day.
- When tincture is ready, strain liquid through muslin cloth, muslin bag, cheesecloth or coffee filter by hand into bowl, or use a tincture press.
- Pour extracted liquid preferably into dark glass dropper bottles.
- At the first sign of a cold, flu or infection, it is important to strengthen immune system. Take 3 squirts or 1 teaspoon every hour the first day and every two hours the second day. Then 3 to 5 times a day for a week or until feeling better.
- Take 3 squirts or 1 teaspoon daily to strengthen immune system.
- Medicinal purposes mentioned or suggested throughout book.

Lip Balm

Ingredients:
- 2 ounces any carrier oil. Use 1 kind of oil or mix 2 carrier oils at 1 ounce each such as almond, argan, coconut, emu, extra virgin olive, grapeseed, hemp, jojoba, safflower, sesame or sunflower.
- 1 ounce beeswax (vegan alternative is carnauba wax).

Optional:
- Flavoring suggestions are 1 teaspoon of lip balm flavoring, 1 teaspoon of vanilla extract or 5 to 10 drops of essential oils like clary sage, geranium, lavender, peppermint, rose or wintergreen.
- Coloring suggestions are adding a piece of natural eye shadow or lipstick, ½ teaspoon of alkanet root powder or beet powder.
- Preservative suggestions are a few drops of vitamin E oil or grapefruit seed extract.
- Use previously prepared herbal oil or make and use herbal oil instead of plain carrier oil using herbs such as echinacea, lavender, myrrh or peppermint.

How to Make
- Heat carrier oil or herbal oil and melt beeswax together in small crock-pot.
- Turn off heat and allow to cool slightly before filling containers.
- Stir in flavoring, color and/or preservative at this point.
- Fill about twenty lip tubes, small tins or jars.
- Optional to use lip tube filling tray and transfer pipettes.

- Allow to cool and harden.

Menthol Salve

Ingredients:
- 4 ounces extra virgin olive oil or make and use previously prepared herbal oil. Herb suggestions include cayenne, comfrey, eucalyptus, lavender, medical marijuana, mullein, peppermint or St. John's Wort

1 ounce of each:
- Menthol crystals
- Beeswax (vegan alternative is carnauba wax)

1 teaspoon of each:
- Birch essential oil
- Peppermint essential oil
- Eucalyptus essential oil
- Wintergreen essential oil

How to Make & Use
- Heat extra virgin olive oil or herbal oil, menthol crystals and melt beeswax in small crock-pot.
- Turn off heat, let cool a bit and add essential oils.
- Stir to blend; put warm liquid salve into jars to harden. If using plastic containers, be careful oil is not too hot or your containers could melt.
- Start by filling only one jar to harden to test the consistency of salve. If too hard, put back into crock-pot and add some extra virgin olive oil; if it is too loose, add some more wax. Caution - keep away from eyes.
- Some uses include sore muscles, decongestant, sunburn and headaches.
- Medicinal purposes mentioned or suggested throughout book.

Mouthwash

Ingredients:
- 25 to 40 ounces distilled water
- ¼ to ½ cup of xylitol powder
- 2 to 3 ounces of food grade peroxide or can use 3% peroxide
- 3 to 7 drops grapefruit seed extract
- 5 to 10 drops essential oils of your choice like birch, cinnamon, clove, fennel, lemon, myrrh, oregano, peppermint, sage, spearmint or tea tree

1 ounce of each:
- Himalayan sea salt powder or sole water
- Colloidal silver

How to Make & Use
- Whisk ingredients together in a bowl before pouring into bottle(s), or add ingredients into a bottle and shake well to blend.
- Gargle 1 to 2 tablespoons once or twice a day for about a minute or two. Swish through teeth, open wide and gargle to get to back of mouth; spit out.
- Use after brushing teeth, flossing, tongue cleaning or oil pulling.
- Helps reduce gum pain, plaque on teeth, dry mouth and bacteria in mouth.

Powder

Ingredients - 1 cup each of:
- Arrowroot powder
- Baking soda
- Bentonite clay
- Corn starch
- Optional to add 5 to 10 drops of essential oils like chamomile, geranium, lavender or rose

Mix ingredients together; break up any lumps with a fork, or put in blender for a few seconds. Store in closed container or shaker bottle.

Salt Scrub - use 1 to 2 times a week.

Ingredients:
- ½ cup fine Himalayan sea salt.
- 1 to 2 tablespoons ground apricot kernels or ground almonds; ground in mortar & pestle or blender.
- 2 to 3 tablespoons any warmed carrier oil such as almond, argan, coconut, emu, grapeseed, hemp, jojoba, safflower, sesame or sunflower.
- 2 to 5 drops of lavender essential oil.

How to Make & Use
- Mix ingredients together in a bowl.
- Rub on skin gently for about 5 to 10 minutes.
- Rinse off with warm water or shower off.
- Use on face or body to improve circulation, cleanse skin and remove dead skin cells.
-

Sanitizing Oil

Ingredients:

- 1 ounce coconut oil.
- 1 teaspoon sole water (see Himalayan Sea Salt).
- 5 to 7 drops grapefruit seed extract.
- 5 drops each of oregano & tea tree essential oils.

How to Make & Use
- Mix ingredients together in any jar with a lid.
- Some uses include hand sanitizer or apply to cuts, scrapes and rashes.

Sports/Electrolyte Drink
Ingredients:
- ¼ to 1 teaspoon Himalayan sea salt or sole water.
- ¼ cup aloe vera juice.
- 1 tablespoon baking soda.
- Squeeze in juice of 1 to 2 whole lemons and/or limes.
- 1 to 3 tablespoons raw honey or flavored stevia extract.

Mix ingredients together in 16 ounce bottle; then fill with filtered water, distilled water or coconut water.

Sunscreen Oil
Ingredients:
- 2 ounces red raspberry seed oil.
- 1 ounce avocado oil.
- 1 ounce wheat germ oil.
- 10 to 20 drops carrot seed essential oil.
- 5 to 10 drops lavender essential oil.

How to Make & Use
- Mix ingredients together in a 4 ounce bottle.
- You will need to reapply oil about every 1 to 2 hours.
- Also a good daily face & neck moisturizing oil.
- Optional to add 1 tablespoon of zinc oxide pharmaceutical grade powder, use with caution.
- Stay away from citrus essential oils, which have been known to burn the skin while in the sun.

Oils and butters that are known to contain sun blocking protection:
- Avocado Oil
- Cocoa Butter
- Hazelnut Oil
- Red Raspberry Seed Oil
- Rosehip Oil
- Shea Butter

- Hemp Oil
- Jojoba Oil
- Pomegranate Seed Oil
- Virgin Coconut Oil
- Walnut Oil
- Wheat Germ Oil

Essential oils that are known to contain sun blocking protection:
- Carrot Seed
- Chamomile
- Eucalyptus
- Helichrysum
- Lavender
- Myrrh

Super Tonic

Grind ingredients in blender:
- ½ cup ginger root
- ½ cup horseradish root
- 1 whole small onion
- 1 whole bulb of peeled garlic cloves
- 1 to 3 cayenne, jalapeno or habanero peppers
- ½ to 1 cup apple cider vinegar
- Optional - ½ cup turmeric root

How to Make & Use
- Fill canning jars or glass jars with lids about ⅓ full with ground vegetable mush. Then fill jars with apple cider vinegar.
- Cover and keep jars on counter, in cabinet or in refrigerator. Shake every day for 2 weeks, then strain. Optional to leave in vegetables.
- Store in the refrigerator & will last for years.
- At the first sign of a cold, flu or infection, important to strengthen immune system. Take 3 squirts or 1 teaspoon every hour the first day and every two hours the second day. Then 3 to 5 times a day for a week or until better.
- Take 1 teaspoon daily to strengthen immune system.
- Sore throat - take 1 tablespoon straight and/or gargle 1 teaspoon for about 30 to 60 seconds; spit out.
- Heartburn or coughing - take 1 tablespoon straight, followed by a glass of water.
- Tea - by adding 1 to 3 tablespoons to cup of hot water.
- Use as a salad dressing or marinade.

Take 1 teaspoon to 1 tablespoon Super Tonic daily to:
- Help strengthen immune system.
- Improve heartburn and digestion.
- Helps fight against colds, flu and sinus issues.

- Helps remove heavy metals, yeast and parasites.
- Benefits the heart, liver, kidneys and colon.

Throat Gargle

Ingredients:
- 1 cup of herbal tea. Herb suggestions include green tea, mullein, sage and peppermint; use fresh, dried or powdered herbs.
- 1 to 2 dashes hot sauce or ¼ to ½ teaspoon of cayenne pepper powder
- Juice of half lemon.

1 tablespoon of each:
- Apple cider vinegar.
- Himalayan sea salt powder or sole water.
- Raw honey.

How to Make & Use
- While herbal tea is still warm, wisk all ingredients together in a bowl, pour into bottle(s) and store in the refrigerator.
- Sore throat - gargle 1 tablespoon for about 30 to 60 seconds; spit out. Gargle every half hour to an hour the first day and then every couple
- hours for few days or until better.

Tooth Powder - is known to kill bacteria, whiten teeth & reduce plaque.

Ingredients - 1 tablespoon of each:
- Baking soda
- Bentonite clay
- Coral calcium powder
- Himalayan sea salt powder
- Xylitol powder
- Activated charcoal powder
- Optional to add 1 to 3 drops of an essential oil like cinnamon, clove, fennel, myrrh, orange, oregano, peppermint, spearmint or sweet basil.

How to Make & Use
- Mix ingredients together and put powder mixture into small jars so that each person will have their own. Dampen toothbrush, dip in jar and brush.

DIY RECIPES FOR CLEANING PRODUCTS

These are ideas & suggestions. You can change or adjust as you need or desire.

All-purpose Cleaners
1. Mix together in 8 ounce spray bottle - 7 ounces of water and 1 ounce natural dish soap, liquid castile soap, *Miracle II* soap or your favorite natural liquid soap.
2. Mix together in 16 ounce spray bottle - cup of water & cup of white vinegar, apple cider vinegar or 3% hydrogen peroxide. Optional to add a few squirts of natural dish soap, liquid castile soap, *Miracle II* soap or your favorite natural liquid soap.
3. Borax spray - in a bowl, whisk together 2 cups of hot water with ¼ cup borax & juice of whole lemon. Allow to cool before pouring into spray bottle.

Optional to add to any all-purpose cleaner:
- 8 to 15 drops of essential oils like lavender, lemon, lime, pine, rosemary, tea tree or thyme.
- Citrus peels or fresh herb leaves such as eucalyptus, lavender or rosemary.

Coffee Pot Shake
Ingredients:
- Coffee pot filled halfway with ice cubes
- ½ cup any salt
- Cut up lemon

Put ingredients in coffee pot; shake ice mixture to loosen stains and rinse out.

Drain Cleaner
- Pour ½ cup baking soda down drain.
- Follow with 1 cup of white vinegar or 3% hydrogen peroxide.
- Allow to foam for 10 minutes & optional to cover.
- Pour down ½ gallon to 1 gallon of boiling water.
- Finish by running hot water for a minute.
- Helps to snake drain before and after.

Dryer Sheets

Ingredients:

- ½ cup white vinegar or apple cider vinegar
- ½ cup natural fabric softener
- Optional to add 10 to 20 drops of lavender essential oil

How to Make & Use

- Cut up plain colorless fabric, old shirt or muslin cloth into about 6 inch by 6 inch squares.
- Mix ingredients together in a bowl, moisten squares and squeeze most liquid from squares.
- Lay moist squares out to dry and keep dried squares in a closed container.
- Add 1 to 2 squares to dryer per load.

Glass Cleaner

Ingredients:

- 1 cup white vinegar
- 1 cup distilled water or any water
- 8 to 15 drops any citrus essential oil of choice

Pour ingredients into 16 ounce spray bottle; shake to blend.

Laundry Detergent

Ingredients - 1 cup each:

- Baking soda
- Borax
- *Oxi-Clean* (preferably *Oxi-Clean free)*
- Washing soda

Mix ingredients together and store in closed container. Use ½ to 1 cup per average load.

Scouring Powder

Ingredients - ¼ cup of each:

- Any salt
- Baking soda
- Bentonite clay or food grade diatomaceous earth
- Borax

Mix ingredients together and keep in a shaker jar.

Toilet Bowl Cleaner

Ingredients:
- ¼ to ½ cup baking soda or borax
- ¼ to ½ cup of white vinegar or 3% hydrogen peroxide

Put ingredients into toilet and scrub.

Resources

Batmanghelidj, F. MD. *You're Not Sick, You're Thirsty* (Warner Books, 2003)

Balch, Phyllis A. *Prescription for Nutritional Healing* (Penguin Group, 2006)

Carter, Mildred & Weber, Tammy. *Body Reflexology* (Parker publishing, 1994)

Clark, Ph.D., Hulda Regehr. *The Cure for All Diseases* (ProMotion Publishing, 1995)

Cornett, James W. *How Indians Used Desert Plants* (Nature Trails Press, 2002)

Evans, Mark B. Phil. *Yoga, Tai Chi, Massage and Healing Remedies* (Anness Publishing Ltd., 2002)

Hale, Gill. *The Practical Encyclopedia of Feng Shui* (Hermes House, 2004)

Hall, Judy. *The Crystal Bible* (Godsfield Press, 2003)

Jarvis, D.C. *Folk Medicine* (Fawcett Publications, Inc., 1958)

Keith, Velma J. & Gordon, Monteen. *The How to Herb Book* (Rosehaven Publishing, 1984)

Kirschner, H. E., M.D. *Nature's Healing Grasses* (H. C. White Publications)

Kushi, Michio. *Your face Never Lies* (Red Moon Press, 1976)

Mojay, Gabriel. *Aromatherapy for Healing the Spirit* (Healing Arts Press, 1997)

Marquardt, Hanne. *Reflex Zone Therapy of the Feet* (Healing Arts Press, 1984)

Mills, Linn & Post, Dick. *Nevada Gardener's Guide* (Cool Springs Press, 2005)

Moore, Michael. *Medicinal Plants of the Desert and Canyon West* (Museum of New Mexico Press, 1989)

Ohashi with Tom Monte. *Reading the Body* (Penguin Group, 1991)

O'Shea,Tim. *The Sanctity of Human Blood: Vaccination is Not Immunization* (New West 2000)

Richards, Carol. *Take a Break Self Meditate* (Balboa Press, 2013)

Ritchason N.D. Jack. *The Little Herb Encyclopedia* (Woodland Health Books, 1995)

Rhode, David. *Native Plants of Southern Nevada* (The University of Utah Press, 2002)

Rose, Jeanne. *Herbs and Things* (Grosset & Dunlap Workman Publishing, 1979)

Rose, Jeanne. *The Aromatherapy Book* (North Atlantic Books, 1992)

Royal, Penny C. *Herbally Yours* (Sound Nutrition, 1982)

Salaman, Maureen. *Foods That Heal* (Statford Publishing, 1989)

Sweet, Muriel. *Common Edible and Useful Plants of the West* (Naturegraph Publishers, Inc., 1975)

Tilford, Gregory L. *Edible and Medicinal Plants of the West* (Mountain Press Publishing Co., 1997)

White M.D., Linda B. & Foster, Steven. *The Herbal Drugstore* (Rodale Inc., 2000)

Wormwood, Susan & Valerie Ann. *Essential Aromatherapy* (New World Library, 1995)